"99+ Healings And Cures You Have To Know And More!"

"99+ Healings And Cures You Have To Know And More!"

UPDATED: 252334C February 2019

Published By Joseph A. Laydon Jr.

Website: https://www.survivalexpertblog.com

E-Mail: wwwsurvivalexpert@yahoo.com

MOST IMPORTANT NOTE: The individual *"99+ Healings And Cures You Have To Know And More!"* is a compilation from my already published Anytime Anywhere Survival Newsletters (AASNs) and the *Gettysburg Program* at http://www.survivalexpert.com

Published By Joseph A. Laydon Jr.

Website: https://www.survivalexpertblog.com

Copyright & Disclaimer

IRISAP DISCLAIMER STATEMENT

Table Of Contents

Contents

Dedication!

This Book is dedicated to all the hard-working medical practitioners who work in the many alternative healthcare practices across the United States and across the globe.

This Book is also dedicated to all the patients on the receiving end of alternative healthcare practices. Thank you for BELIEVING in many Alternative Healthcare Practices.

This Book is also dedicated to all the lawyers defending healtcare practitioners who are being sued by plaintiffs supporting conventional medicine.

Introduction!

Welcome to *"99+ Alternative Healings And Cures You Have To Know And More!"*

Welcome and thank you for getting *"99+ Alternative Healings And Cures You Have To Know And More!"* where you'll find real applications to fight minor to serious maladies.

"99+ Alternative Healings And Cures You Have To Know And More!" is an Introduction to **'More Super Healthy Survival Books Just For You'** *found at at the end of this Survival Book.*

Somebody in your family household has to be the Survival Expert – even when it comes fighting minor to severe killer maladies when absolutely no professional medical assistance is available. Somebody has to be the Survival Expert, why not you? And here's a good start so you're ready Anytime Anywhere!

Again, thank you for getting this Book. I welcome you forwarding and concerns with respect to this Book.

IMPORTANT NOTE: I attempted to put all these *"99+ Alternative Healings And Cures You Have To Know And More!"* in perfect alphabetical order but several applications matched or complimented each other. I encourage you to read this Survival Book multiple times so *You're Ready Anytime Anywhere!*

99+ Alternative Healings And Cures You Have To Know And More!

We all are vulnerable to minor to severe maladies that will eventually have us all leave this Earth. However, your amazing body has the innate ability to heal itself. You just have to give it a *'kick in the butt'* to get the healing process started. This Survival Book is dedicated to alternative methods towards the healing process. Let's start with *Amazing Gua Sha Detox*.

Amazing Gua Sha Detox: Gua Sha is an ancient Chinese therapy that's been practiced by the Chinese for thousands of years. Gua Sha focuses on one thing - it helps detoxify your body. Its main purpose is to detoxify your body which in turns helps remedy many common maladies and improve vitality.

Gua Sha therapist use a thin hard flat-like tool about the size of a fist (03 1/2-inches by 02-inches). It's scraped over the biggest organ of the body - the skin. The back and forth scraping friction motion over the oiled skin brings the toxins to the skin's surface thus leaving the body. The Gua Sha tool is scraped over the entire surface of the body. One treatment takes about 10 - 20 minutes.

Gua Sha Therapy is known to help alleviate, remedy, eliminate and or improve arthritis, asthma, energy, fatigue, headaches, lethargy, mental clarity, skin problems,...

A single Gua Sha treatment cost about $100 and to get the full effect of Gua Sha Therapy, it takes about 08 treatments.

According to happy recipients of Gua Sha Therapy, the price is well worth the results! Look in your local phone book for a Gua Sha Therapist nearest you and get DETOXED!

Note: Insure you seek advice from your doctor prior to implementing any alternative therapy or adding or deleting and foods, supplements to your current diet.

Amish Cancer Flushers: Here are the foods that help flush carcinogens (cancer-causing agents) out of your body and fight specific cancers:

a) Beans---------------------colon cancer
b) Beet----------------------cervical cancer
c) Blackberry Tea-----------general
d) Broccoli-----------------general
e) Brussels Sprouts---------general
f) Cabbage------------------general
g) Carrots------------------colon cancer
h) Cauliflower-------------breast cancer & general
i) Chives-------------------stomach cancer
j) Garlic-------------------stomach & colon cancer
k) Leeks--------------------stomach cancer
l) Onions-------------------stomach cancer & general
m) Pear---------------------colon cancer
n) Radishes-----------------general
o) Shallots----------------stomach cancer
p) Spinach------------------lung cancer & general
q) Sweet Potato-------------general
r) Tomatoes-----------------stomach, pancreatic & general

s) Vitamin C----------------mouth, esophagus &
                            stomach cancers
See *Cancer Hospitals & Clinics That Offer Alternative Therapies*.

If you don't know about Jerry Baker, you will by the time you finish this segment. I've purchased several very informative products from Jerry Baker and I highly recommend ANY of his products. All of Jerry Baker's tips are time-proven and really work and these tips come from one of his latest publications - *"Grandma Putt's Old-Time Vinegar, Garlic, Baking Soda, And 101 More Problem Solvers!"* and other publications (see *Jerry Baker* in POC Section). The following tips are orientated towards healing-up your body. Let's get started with *Baker's All Body Itch Remedy*.

Baker's All Body Itch Remedy: If you're all ate up with insect bites, poison ivy rashes or sunburn all over you body, it can surely be non-stop itching torture. You need to submerge your entire body in warm water. A full cup of salt added to the warm water will aid to stop the itch. If you have an ocean nearby, take a long dip in shallow salt water.

1st Note: Upon completing SERE Instructor Course located in Fort Sherman, Panama - less than half the class survived (met course standards) to graduate. Upon being extracted from the Panamanian jungle, accounting for equipment, and debriefed, we were all seen by the doctor and weighed-in. I lost 25-pounds the last week while the average weight-loss was about 20-pounds through the evasion and isolation phase.

Anyway, we all had one thing in common, we were all ate up real bad with insect bites of all types from the top of our heads to the bottom of our feet. Some had it real bad having a bite every square inch of their body.

But we were all in such bad condition (physically & mentally), I don't even remember feeling any itching at any time. I remember our hands having hundreds of small cuts from the black palm and felt no pain because of our incapacitated state. The doc prescribed Benedryl and multiple dips in the salty Atlantic Ocean very nearby.

2nd Note: Upon negotiating and completing US Army Ranger School, I recollect seeing my hands all cut and scraped-up but felt no pain. Why? I figure it was the very poor physical and mental condition at the time. I guess the body probably shut down the pain sensors to the hands to prioritize on other parts of the body.

Baker's Athlete's Foot Remedy: Apple cider vinegar will help remedy your Athletes foot. Just apply it several times a day and you'll be back on your feet in no time.

Baker's Cramp Packets: Are you feeling a cramp coming on. Muscle cramps no matter where they're located in your body hurt awful bad. And leg cramps will literally stop you in your tracks and like I said before, if you become immobile in a wilderness environment, you're trapped in a potentially killer environment - you're in the food-chain and some critter(s) got you on their dinner table.

Next time you visit a fast food restaurant, grab
several mustard packets and put them in your backpack
(in their own container). When you feel muscle cramps
coming on, swallow the contents of a mustard packet and
chase it with a full cup of fresh pure water. This
concoction will aid to stop muscle cramps in their
tracks.

Baker's Pain & Itch Remedy: Insects of all sorts will
bite into you or insert stingers into you. In either
case they cause pain, itching, and swelling. As soon
as possible, dab the bite or sting site with some
vinegar so to neutralize the poison. If time has
passed, still dab the site with vinegar to relieve the
pain and itching.

Baker's Poison Neutralizer: Neutralize the poison of
insect bites, jelly fish stings,... and you prevent or
stop the pain, swelling and itching. Just take a pinch
of meat tenderizer, add a little water or your own
spit, mix it into a paste and apply it to the site(s).

Baker's Poison Plant Remedy: When venturing outdoors,
many times you can't avoid poisonous plants like poison
ivy, poison oak, poison sumac, stinging nettles, common
ivy,... To remedy the non-stop itch from contact
dermatitis, make a concoction of equal parts apple
cider vinegar and fresh water. Dab this concoction on
the itchy sites and you should find relief real soon.

Baker's Rehydration: Dehydration in a wilderness environment is inviting killer trouble with open arms.

Believe me - when you're dehydrated, your mental functions are out the window. You're lethargic and you don't care anymore. You have to get rehydrated and NOW! Here's Jerry Baker's rehydration concoction. Mix 01 quart of fresh pure water with 01 teaspoon of salt and 04 teaspoons of sugar. Drink 02 cups of this concoction every hour till your able to think straight again!

Brussels Sprouts: One-half cup of raw Brussels Sprouts provide only twenty calories while one-half cup of cooked Brussels sprouts provides 30 calories. A member of the cruciferous vegetable family (broccoli, cabbage, cauliflower), Brussels Sprouts can fill you up and help you lose weight.

A cooked cup of this tasty treat is rich in Vitamin C, provides a good share of Vitamin A, iron, potassium, riboflavin, and rich in protein. Brussels Sprouts are very low in fat and sodium and provide fiber.

<u>Brussels Sprouts are a good bet to inhibit cancer, especially colon and stomach cancer</u>. According to Dr. Saxon Graham's 1978 study in Buffalo, New York, Brussels sprouts emerged (along with cabbage and broccoli) as outstanding in saving lives from colon cancer!

According to a study in Norway, eating more cruciferous vegetables, _including Brussels Sprouts, may suppress the precancerous growths in the colon called polyps in which cancer initially surfaces_. Brussels Sprouts and other cruciferous vegetables may also cut the risk of bladder, esophageal, lung, rectal, stomach and rectal cancer!

Brussels Sprouts Tasty Recipe!

MOST IMPORTANT NOTE: Here's my quick very tasty recipe for Brussels Sprouts. I normally don't eat or like the taste of Brussels Sprouts till I cooked em' up like I do in this recipe.

Ingredients: 24 Brussels Sprouts, sharp knife, frying pan, coconut oil, bowl, fork, sea salt, and wooden spoon.

Step 01: Take a frying pan put it on one of your burners at medium heat.

Step 02: Immediately spoon-out 05 good oversized scoops of coconut oil (will be semi-solid at room temperature) and put them in the frying pan and wait till the coconut oil starts sizzle.

Step 03: Procure 24 Brussels Sprouts and cut off the base (stalk) of each of them. Then remove 03 or 04 outer leaves (debris) and place them in the frying pan.

Step 04: Every couple minutes, or so, gently stir the Brussels Sprouts in the frying pan with your wooden spoon till they are all golden brown.

Step 05: Remove to Brussels Sprouts to a bowl and sprinkle them with sea salt. Fork-in and enjoy with a cold bottle of beer.

Note: I tried cooking the Brussels Sprouts with other oils, but coconut oil is the tastiest and it's a Medium-Chain Triglyceride (MTC) meaning it helps you burn fat far better than other oils that aren't MTCs.

1st Coma Remedy: Coma is a physical state when the body is unresponsive to external stimuli. Coma is often induced to perform very delicate surgical operations or when the body is seriously damaged. On 22 February 2008, it was reported that a man brought his wife out of her coma. How? He yelled at her! Many unconscious patients are talked to by their caretakers (nurses, family friends,...). It is noted that talking to unconscious patients has healing benefits. So why not yell at patients in a state of coma? Heck, it works when Drill Instructors are yelling at bonehead, know-nuthin privates in Basic Training!

2nd Coma Remedy: Every now and then I listen to the Bob & Tom Show on FM radio. One morning (08 May 2009) they had a comedian & actor guest on their show by the name - I believe - Tom Wilson. He starred as Biff in the *Back To The Future* movies. Anyway, he related how he helped a man come out of a coma. He stated he got an amazing e-mail from a man in Scotland.

The man was in a coma. His family knew he liked *Back To The Future* movies and thought they might help him out. The family played the movies and sure enough, he came out of his coma!!!

Note: There is definitely something about the human voice. To prove this point, what does your favorite music do to your mood, your emotions,... Better yet, how about a human voice that eventually built a movement and a war machine the world had never known at the time. A voice that was instrumental in the deaths of millions.

His name is Adolf Hitler and has gone down in history as the most evil human in human history. Enough -

Cabbage Bandage Remedy: Approximately 15 December 2011 (Thursday) I woke-up with my right knee in pain that ached 24-hours a day non-stop. From what I can tell, directly over the kneecap was a "bubble" of liquid the size of a 50 cent piece. Water on the knee??? Anyway, the pain progressed where it was even difficult to sleep. Then on the evening of 18 December 2011 (Sunday) I took action.

There are hundreds of remedies in this Survival Program but I wanted to add another. So I went to this website I gave you years ago - www.earthclinic.com I went there a read about the additional amazing benefits of cabbage - namely joint pain. I modified what I read and here it is:

Ingredients: Fresh head of green cabbage, small plastic bag and bandage wrap.

Step 01: Take the fresh head of green cabbage and tear away and discard the first few outer leaves (debris, discolored,…)

Step 02: Carefully tear away 05 or 06 large leaves.

Step 03: Remove any large stalks on any of the leaves so you end-up with pliable cabbage leaves.

Step 04: Place all the pliable leaves in the plastic bag and secure the opening of the bag.

Step 05: Gently roll the cabbage leaves against themselves so bruising is caused so to release their healing ingredients.

Step 06: Remove the cabbage leaves from the plastic bag and place them directly on the injured part of the joint. The cabbage leaves can be placed one on top of the other (which is what I did) or spread to cover the entire circumference of the joint.

Step 07: Secure the cabbage leaves by wrapping the bandage with several snug but NOT TIGHT wraps. The *cabbage bandage* should be applied prior to going to sleep.

What you just read is exactly what I did. I woke-up the next morning (Monday) and was very surprised that there was great improvement. My knee wasn't 100% but the pain was 95% gone and mobility about 80%. I did not reapply the cabbage bandage but as the days went on, my right knee kept improving. The kneecap area is still tender to the touch but overall, the cabbage bandage did the trick.

UPDATE: 02 months later, my knee is in 100% working order thanks to the Cabbage Bandage Remedy. Cabbage deserves more "intensive research."

UPDATE UPDATE: As I update this segment for this Survival Book (23 October 2018 - Tuesday), that NON-STOP PAIN on my right knee never returned all these years (almost 07-years ago) and my knee has always been 100% in working order.

Canadian Diabetes Cure: According to a Canadian study, approximately *"40% of Type 2 diabetes patients can regain normal insulin production and go off their meds in four months! And it reverses prediabetes, too."* The Canadian study discovered the patient must:

- **Drop Weight:** Losing just 05% of your body weight brings down diabetes markers as much as diabetes medications. And for prediabetes patients, losing 05% - 07% of your body weight lowers your diabetes risks by 54%. Losing the weight lowers multi-organ resistance to insulin and gets the pancreas to produce more insulin.

- **Drink A Little Wine:** Drinking just 05-ounces of wine 04 or 05 times a week lowers the risk of diabetes by 58%. The wine slows down the liver's glucose production. Beer and hard liquor are not options. Drink wine.

- **Eat Fresh Fruit:** Eating fiber-rich fresh fruits like pears and oranges on a daily basis, reduces the risk of diabetes by 12%. The fiber in the fruit slows down the absorption of sugars into the bloodstream.
- **Exercise For 10-Minutes:** A 10-minute walk after each meal cuts down the risk of Type 2 Diabetes by 30%. See *U.S. Army Rifle Drill Exercises (07)*.

Cancer Hospitals & Clinics That Offer Alternative Therapies: Here's a list of clinics that are beyond the borders of the United States that offer alternative health practices that are banned in the United States.

Name Of Hospitals / Clinics   **Location**

- Almater Hospital-------------------Mexico
- Angeles Functional Oncology---------Mexico
- Balboa Hospital--------------------Mexico
- CHIPSA Hospital--------------------Mexico
- Galenia Hospital-------------------Mexico
- Gerson Clinic----------------------Mexico
- Hospital Angeles-------------------Mexico
- Hospital Country 2000--------------Mexico
- Hospital De La Familia-------------Mexico
- Hospital San Jose Tec De Monterrey--Mexico
- Hospital Velmar--------------------Mexico
- Integrative Whole Health Clinic-----Mexico
- International Bio Care-------------Mexico
- Issels Integrative Immuno-Oncology—Mexico

- Oasis Of Hope----------------------Mexico
- San Angel Hospital-----------------Mexico
- Sanoviv Medical Institute----------Mexico
- Stella Maris Clinic----------------Mexico

See *The Hoxsey Story* towards the end of this Book.

Cannabis Cancer Healer: Here's a powerful alternative medicine that made a believer out of me. Well before I did my *"intensive research"* I already knew there was something to cannabis healing cancer but my research ordered me to add it to this book to insure you know the real deal about this healing wonder, so here it goes.

A website called ProCon.org (History Timeline Medical Marijuana) does an excellent job in giving the history of cannabis. But here's a brief brief segment for you.

As far back as 2,900 BC, Chinese Emperor named Fu Hsi referred to Ma (cannabis) as a <u>popular medicine</u> that possessed both yin and yang (02 forces of the universe which yin is the passive negative force and yang the active positive force).

Our first President – George Washington, grew hemp for 30-years on his plantation at Mount Vernon, Virginia from 1745 to 1775. In his diary, George Washington had interest with growing his cannabis which had a high THC (Tetrahydrocannabinol) content.

In 1964, Dr. Raphael Mechoulam, Professor of Medicinal Chemistry at the Hebrew University of Jerusalem was the 1st to discover THC (Tetrahydrocannabinol) the main psychoactive ingredient of cannabis. Dr. Mechoulam is also the 1st to synthesize THC.

In 1978, New Mexico was the 1st state to recognize the medicinal use of marijuana. Below is a list of all 30 states that have legalized the medicinal use of marijuana and other uses.

In 1980, a synthetic version of THC (Tetrahydrocannabinol) called Marinol and marijuana was tested on cancer patients. Overall, more patients favored real marijuana as their choice to remedy their cancer over Marinol. However, the US Government gave the GO to Marinol over natural marijuana. In May 1985, Marinol was approved by the FDA (Food & Drug Administration).

On 05 November 1996, California was the 1st state to legalize 'medical marijuana.'

On 07 October 2003, the United States Department of Health and Human Services receives a patent (US 6,630,507 B1) for the therapeutic use of "cannabinoids as antioxidants and neuroprotectants."

On 18 December 2004, an AARP (American Association of Retired Persons) poll found that 72% of seniors support the use of medical marijuana.

In September 2008, 02-pounds of packaged marijuana was found in a Chinese tomb that was 2,700 years old.

In November 2011, a study found that the use of medical marijuana reduced car accidents by 9%. Why? Because drivers were smoking their marijuana versus drinking alcohol when driving.

THC (Tetrahydrocannabinol) in cannabis oil may be the trick to fight and beat cancer but there may be another angle to it. Cannabis Oil induces apoptosis. It gets cancer cells to commit suicide. It gets cancer cells to self-destruct.

States And US Territories Legalizing Medicinal Marijuana And Other Uses!

Number	Date	State
01	05 November 1996	California
02	03 November 1998	Alaska
03	03 November 1998	Oregon
04	03 November 1998	Washington
05	02 November 1999	Maine
06	14 June 2000	Hawaii
07	07 November 2000	Colorado
08	07 November 2000	Nevada
09	26 May 2004	Vermont
10	02 November 2004	Montana
11	03 January 2006	Rhode Island
12	13 March 2007	New Mexico
13	04 November 2008	Michigan
14	11 January 2010	New Jersey
15	27 July 2010	Washington D.C.
15	02 November 2010	Arizona
16	13 May 2011	Delaware
17	31 May 2012	Connecticut
18	06 November 2012	Massachusetts
19	23 July 2013	New Hampshire
20	01 August 2013	Illinois
21	14 April 2014	Maryland
22	29 May 2014	Minnesota
23	05 July 2014	New York
24	03 May 2015	Puerto Rico
25	17 April 2016	Pennsylvania

Number	Date	State
26	17 April 2016	West Virginia
27	08 June 2016	Ohio
28	08 November 2016	Florida
29	08 November 2016	Arkansas
30	08 November 2016	North Dakota
31	10 January 2017	Guam

Note: Each state and territory has their own specific laws with respect to purchasing, possession, cultivation, quantity,… of marijuana and marijuana derivatives. See your local attorney and police for marijuana in your state.

Capsicum (cayenne): Herbal parts are taken from berries and fruits. It acts as a catalyst for herbs and provides apsaicine, capsacutin, capsaicin, capsanthine, capsico, PABA, Vitamins A, B1, B2, B3, B5, B6, B9, C (rich source), E, ascorbic acid, calcium, dihydrocapsaicin, homocapsaicin, homodihydrocapsaicin, iron, magnesium, phosphorus, potassium, selenium, sulphur, and zinc.

Capsicum is the source of over 100 varieties of Cayenne Pepper, from heat ranges of mild paprika to the extremely hot habanera. It's been used for medicinal purposes for thousands of years!

Capsicum aids digestion, <u>improves circulation</u>, and stops bleeding from ulcers. It is noted to also be good for the kidneys, lungs, spleen, pancreas, heart and stomach. It's also noted to help remedy chronic fatigue, depression, gastric ulcers, and prostration. Skin ointments that contain capsaicin have been noted to significantly relieve the pain of arthritis, herpes zoster, and diabetic neuropathy (causes pain and tingling in the legs).

Capsaicin is noted to deplete Substance-P, a neuropeptide produced by the nerves that carry pain sensation. You'll find many new pain-relieving products on the market containing capsicum-capsaicin! Most herbalists have noted that cayenne pepper stops bleeding!

Below is a list of capsicum and their measurements in Scoville Heat Units (SHU). Most actual cayenne pepper is rated between 30,000 to 80,000 Scoville Heat Units. Cayenne just refers to one variety of capsicum. ALL hot peppers are capsicum.

- Paprika - 0 Scoville Heat Units
- Jalapeno - 50,000 to 80,000 Scoville Heat Units
- Serrano - 100,000 Scoville Heat Units
- African Bird - 200,000 Scoville Heat Units
- Mexican Habaneros - 250,000 to 300,000 Scoville Heat Units (HOT!!!)

Researchers in Great Britain and Japan have found that cayenne can cause the body to burn up to 25% more calories in a day than it normally would!

Cayenne has the ability to deplete a chemical in the pain-transmission nerves known as Substance-P.

Cayenne is being tested as an all-around analgesic-painkiller! According to Thomas Barks, Ph.D., head of the Department of Pharmacology at the University of Arizona Health Sciences Center in Tucson, a single injection of capsaicin fights certain types of chronic pain in guinea pigs for weeks! Rubbing an ointment of capsaicin on the skin actually numbs the pain locally!

The Thais (Thailand) use capsicum chili peppers as a seasoning and as an appetizer with their meals. Their blood is infused with chili pepper compounds several times a day. Thais physicians have for some time credited regular consumption of chili peppers as the reason <u>that thromboembolism (life-threatening blood clots) are rare among Thais compared to Americans!</u>

German researchers as early as 1965 found chili peppers beneficial for the blood as a fibrinolytic (clot-dissolving) stimulant. After more testing, Sukoon Visudhiphan, M.D. and his colleagues at the Siriraj Hospital in Bangkok suggested that the frequent stimulation of the <u>clot-dissolving mechanism</u> by chili peppers helps keep the Thais immune to thromboembolism (life-threatening blood clots)! See *Richard Quinn's Heart Disease Cure*.

Car Jack Headache Cure: A car jack is an automobile tool used for lifting, prying, changing tires,... and unbelievably it was used to cure headaches and nausea. NO, not by beating the casualty but by a tool to control energy. In the late 1930s, German geographer Hansjoachim van der Esch explored eastern Sahara Desert located in Africa. He discovered that the killer sandstorms caused nausea and terrible headaches. Why?

During the sandstorm, billions of sand particles colliding with each other created huge amounts of static electricity, so much that it caused nausea and headaches. It's estimated that during a sandstorm, the static electricity is raised to as high as <u>80 volts per square yard</u> - that's a heck of a lot of static electricity. That's like walking across your carpet, and zapping the door knob or that 9-life critter with a static electrical spark but several hundred times more powerful!

So savvy geographer explorer Each came up with a cure to rid his body of all that static electricity to remedy his sickly nausea and terrible pounding headaches; he hooked himself up to a car jack and dragged it behind him, thus grounding himself while he travelled the vast expanse of the eastern Sahara Desert. Instead of all that excess electricity going into his body causing nausea and pounding non-stop headaches, it went into the ground via the car jack.

So if you're outdoors and you're suffering from headaches, it may mean a built-up of static electricity. Now you know how to remedy it, plus it may be telling you a storm is coming your way.
See *Train Track Healing Treatment*.

Cauliflower: Cauliflower is a bit more costly, but worth it when it comes to your health. One cup of raw cauliflower furnishes only 31 calories, provides a good source of Vitamin C (one cup equals 100% of RDA), low in sodium, and low in fat.

Cauliflower is noted to help flush fat out of your system. Cauliflower is one of the vegetables recognized by the Committee on Diet, Nutrition and Cancer of the National Academy of Sciences as <u>one of the best bets for preventing cancer</u>! Cauliflower has established itself as being <u>high on the list of anticancer vegetables</u>.

A close cousin to cabbage, broccoli, and Brussels sprouts - all of these vegetables are <u>linked to lower cancer rates, especially of the colon, rectum, stomach, and possibly the bladder and prostate</u>. Norwegians who eat their fair share of cauliflower (along with broccoli, Brussels sprouts, & cabbage) have fewer and smaller precancerous polyps of the colon.

According to a study by Dr. Lee Wattenberg, laboratory animals were fed cauliflower and then given powerful carcinogens like nitrosamines. The animals that ate cauliflower did not readily develop cancers as those animals that didn't eat cauliflower.

Clean Yourself Up From The Inside With Amazing Chelation Therapy:

What is Chelation Therapy?

American Board of Chelation Therapy (ABCT) defines chelation therapy as "A form of medical therapy designed to restore cellular homeostasis by the use of metal binding and/or bio-inorganic agents. The proper application of this modality also requires knowledge of nutrition and exercise, as well as expertise in helping to implement other lifestyle changes." The chelation process originated in 1893 with a French - Swiss chemist named Alfred Werner who received the Nobel Prize in 1913 for his work.

Chelation Therapy uses EDTA (Ethylene Diamine Tetraacetic Acid) or other supplements that carry out heavy metals like lead, cadmium and arsenic, as well as other foreign substances from the body. The purpose of chelation is to **increase the flow of blood to the vital organs and tissues of the body by reducing calcium deposits in the arteries and blood vessels**.

Chelating agents are available in over-the-counter formulas that can be taken orally at home or administered intravenously under the supervision of your doctor. Chelation Therapy has been used effectively to treat arteriosclerosis for **over 40 years** in the U.S.

Chelation Therapy works like a **magnet attracting metal shavings!** When administered as an infusion into the blood stream, it removes metals and metal compounds from the body including but not limited to calcium (works against calcium in atherosclerotic pathology).

Is Chelation Therapy considered nutritional therapy?
Chelation Therapy helps vital nutrients like carbohydrates, enzymes, fats, hormones, minerals, proteins, Vitamins and other food substances **complete their metabolic actions** in your body. These nutrients also help detoxify your body. Chelation Therapy **helps increase the amount of needed oxygen used at the** **_CELLULAR LEVEL_**!

Over 75 trillion cells in your body need oxygen among other elements to function, thus **_HEALING AT THE_** **_CELLULAR LEVEL_** instead of treating symptoms with drugs! Again, each one of those 75 trillion cells need oxygen to function properly. Chelation Therapy can **remove plaque from 75,000 miles of blood vessels throughout your entire body!** Chelation Therapy assists the oxygenation process and significantly affects your health and health-related problems for the better. Especially those health-related problems involving the cardiovascular system, nerves and sex organs.

Can Chelation Therapy be considered to avoid amputation?
It is noted that many patients that had **exhausted all traditional forms of treatment for endstage occlusive peripheral arterial disease, were referred to peripheral vascular surgeons for amputation of their gangrenous limb**. Patients turned to certified Chelation Therapist. Chelation Therapy (EDTA) was therapeutic in **reversing ischemia** (cessation of the flow of blood because of a blocked artery).

What types of degenerative diseases can Chelation Therapy ameliorate, control, reverse, prevent or at least ease the symptoms?

Below is a **partial list** of common degenerative diseases:

- Alzheimer's Disease
- Arteriosclerosis
- Arthritis
- Atherosclerosis
- Cancer
- Cataracts
- Diabetes
- Diabetic Retinopathy
- Digitalis Intoxication
- Gangrene
- Glaucoma
- Heart Arrhythmias
- Heart Attack
- Heavy Metal Poisoning
- High Blood Pressure
- Hypercalcemia
- Impotence
- Kidney Disease
- Intermittent Claudication
- Lupus Erythematosus
- Lou Gehrig's Disease
- Memory
- Multiple Sclerosis
- Macular Degeneration
- And much more!!!

How do I know if Chelation Therapy would benefit me and where can I obtain proper treatment?
Chelation Therapy could probably benefit most people (see your doctor)! The chemical industry admits that **60,000 man-made pollutants have been added to the environment** and Federal estimates suggest another 5,000 substances are intentionally added to food along with another 10,000 pollutants unintentionally included as a result of production or packaging!

It's not uncommon for Chelation Therapy to **improve eyesight!** Chelation Therapy has been successfully used to overcome **cataracts, diabetic retinopathy, glaucoma and macular degeneration!**

Flushing the arteries with IV infusions of EDTA or other IV chelating agents **can bring fresh blood and oxygen to the tissues** and may aid in the healing process!

Health care consumers (YOU) should know about IV Chelation Therapy as an **alternative to coronary artery bypass** and other forms of heart vessel surgery! Most patients suffering from hardening of the arteries generally **receive no information** about alternatives to toxic drugs and dangerous surgery.

How many patients faced with amputation of an arm, foot, hand, or leg because of gangrene, are offered information about an alternative therapy such as Chelation Therapy?

If you have any type of cardiovascular or blood vessel disease or know anyone with a cardiovascular or blood vessel disease, _**consider looking into Chelation Therapy**_.

There are over 150 doctors in the U.S. who are certified by the American Board of Chelation Therapy as approved Chelation Therapist. See *American Board of Chelation Therapy* in the POC Section.

Follow the recommended dosage and instructions from the label and as per your doctor's instructions.

Coenzyme Q10 (CoQ10): CoQ10 was discovered in 1957 by Fred Crane, M.D., from the University of Wisconsin. He isolated CoQ10 from beef hearts. CoQ10 is a Vitamin-like substance that resembles Vitamin E, which may be more powerful as an antioxidant.

Of the 10 common coenzyme Qs, only CoQ10 is found in human tissue. CoQ10 declines with age and should be supplemented in the diet. CoQ10 plays a crucial role in the effectiveness of the immune system and the aging process!

The New England Institute reports that <u>CoQ10 alone is effective in reducing mortality in experimental animals afflicted with tumors and leukemia</u>. <u>It's noted that CoQ10 may be helpful in the complete remission of many cancers</u>!

In Japan, CoQ10 is being used in the treatment of heart disease, high blood pressure and enhance the immune system!

Research has revealed that CoQ10 benefits allergies, asthma, and respiratory disease as well as treating the brain for anomalies of mental function associated with Alzheimer's Disease and schizophrenia. The amazing CoQ10 is also beneficial in aging, candidiasis, diabetes, multiple sclerosis, periodontal disease, and obesity.

AIDS is a primary target for research on CoQ10 because of its immense benefits to the immune system. <u>The use of CoQ10 is a major step forward in the prevention and control of cancer</u>. Use caution when purchasing CoQ10 because not all products are offered in its purest form. CoQ10's natural color is bright yellow\orange and has very little taste in the powdered form. CoQ10 should be kept away from heat and light since pure CoQ10 will deteriorate in temperatures above 115 degrees Fahrenheit.

Sources of CoQ10 are mackerel, salmon, and those tasty sardines. Sardines contain the largest amounts of CoQ10. Authentic CoQ10 can be purchased at many health-food stores.

One study published in the American Journal of Cardiology (1985), 150mg of CoQ10 taken daily by heart patients for 04 weeks reduced the incidence of angina attacks from 5.3 to 2.5 per day. The researchers concluded that CoQ10 actually strengthened the diseased heart, which allowed it to reach higher levels of energy before pain or oxygen deprivation occurs.

In another study published in the American Journal of Cardiology 1990, a long-term study of 126 patients with severe cardiomyopathy that took supplements of CoQ10 prolonged their lives by years, not weeks or months - YEARS! In some patients the disease was eliminated entirely!

Other published studies have noted that <u>CoQ10 helps a wide variety of illnesses, including AIDS, cancer, chronic fatigue, and periodontal disease</u>.

WARNING: To date, no side effects have been documented. Ensure you purchase authentic CoQ10. Some companies put dyes in their fake CoQ10 to achieve the orange color that is found naturally in pure CoQ10! *Follow the recommended dosage and instructions from the label and as per your doctor's instructions.*

Cold Water Cures: If there is one thing I hate more than 08-legged spiders, it's cold frigid water. I can still hold my own when it comes to cold weather to include being soaking wet with cold water (surface or submerged) but I just have a lot of *"Art Of Suffering"* memories (military) when it comes to cold water. Anyway, did you know plain ol' cold water has some very beneficial effects?

According to Gurudev Khar Khalsa, a noted Sat Nam Rasayan Healer and Kundalini Yoga Teacher from Los Angeles, California: *"Cold Water Massage Therapy is one of the healthiest and most inexpensive of therapies. Simply massage the body with almond oil before taking a shower.*

Shower in cold water until your body temperature rises and no longer feels cold, but toasty and warm. Make sure the bathroom is heated. Never get out of a cold shower into a cold room."

And here's list maladies remedied by cold water and complimentary benefits of taking cold showers - Brrrrr:

- Acne
- Allergies
- Anxiety Attacks
- Asthma
- Awake
- Blood Cholesterol Lower
- Blood Circulation
- Blood Pressure Reduced
- Blood Sugar Lowered
- Body Feels Warmer
- Body Odor Eliminated
- Calming Effect
- Cleanses Circulatory System
- Clearer Mind
- Complexion
- Concentration Improvement
- Depression Eliminated
- Dry Skin
- Eliminates Poisons & Toxins
- Energy
- Feelings Of Euphoria
- Five Senses Improved
- Flushes Organs
- Focus Improvement
- Hair Improvement
- Headaches Eliminated

- Heart Problems
- Heightened Awareness
- Immune System Booster
- Learning Improvement
- Less\No Colds
- Less\No Flu
- Leg Bloating\Pain,...
- Libido Improvement
- Mental Faculties Improved
- Migraines Eliminated
- Mood Improvement
- Muscle Cramps
- Pain
- Panic Attacks
- Positive Thoughts
- Pulse Rate Lower
- Rashes
- Refreshed
- Skin Improvement
- Sinusitis
- Sleep Improvement
- Strengthens Nervous System
- Strengthens Mucous Membranes
- Stress Buster
- Sweating Reduced
- Utility Bill Reduced
- Zest For Life

I've told you before that the BLOOD RULES! It's apparent to me that cold showers get the blood moving thus the many benefits of plain ol' *Cold Water Cures!*

Color Therapy: Nobody can deny that different colors affect each of us in different ways and we all have our favorite colors. Pranic Healing uses energy to heal as well as certain colors that have their own specific effects on the body.

Keep this in mind when I talk about the following colors and what they're noted to accomplish for the mind and body. To use the following colors, proper training using various crystals are required**.

Red: Used to help with anemia, bladder infection, circulation, depression, digestion, hypotension, impotence, infertility, lack of energy, forgetfulness, shock,...

Orange: Used to help with allergies, constipation, energy, inhibition, kidney weakness, lactation, muscle cramps, muscle spasms, repression,...

Yellow: Used to help with breathing difficulties, depression, diabetes, digestive problems, food allergies, gallstones, gas, hypoglycemia, hypothyroid, liver problems, mental exhaustion, muscle cramps,...

Blue: Used to help with back pain, burns, colic, digestive irritations, ear infections, fatigue, fever, gum inflammation, hemorrhoids, hyperactive, hypertension, hyperthyroid, inflammations, mentally exhausted, nervousness, skin irritations, skin rashes, sore throat, teething, toxemia of pregnancy, ulcers, vaginal infections,

Green: Used to help with anger, breathing difficulties, <u>cancer</u>, fatigue, heart attack, heart pain, hypertension, insomnia, negativity, paranoia, tension,...

Violet: Used to help with baldness, black eyes, dandruff, depression, migraine headaches, parasites,...

Pink: Used to help with anger, breathing difficulties, <u>cancer</u>, fatigue, heart attack, heart pain, hypertension, insomnia, negativity, paranoia, tension,... See *Prisoner Pink* below.

**Another technique to use if you don't have color crystals is to use Mind-Over-Matter Applications to *"visualize"* that particular color doing its healing on a particular part of the body. See Mind-Over-Matter Applications in this issue under HEALTH.

Color Therapy Application: In this segment we'll use *Color Therapy* to survive in a cold weather environment. I already gave you some good data on Color Therapy and I told you that if you don't have colored crystals, you can use your mind!

The color that we'll use is fire-orange and red which are 02 powerful energy colors! <u>You feel warmer already don't you?</u> Did you see what I just did? I gave you a positive affirmation! OK, let's start. Visualize:

"My underwear are fire-orange that radiate pulses of warm heat no matter if they're dry or soaking wet. My socks are fire-orange that radiate extra heat to my warm feet. My shoes glow from keeping all the extra heat in. All this warm heat is ***KILLING TRILLIONS OF CANCER CELLS.***

My pants, undershirt, shirt, coat, headgear, scarf and gloves are fire-orange that radiate pulsing glowing heat to keep me warm 24-hours a day. And at the same time, the radiating glowing heat is ***KILLING TRILLIONS OF CANCER CELLS.***

41

The glowing fire-orange red is so warm its glow extends beyond my warm body to shield me from cold winds, rain,... I feel the warm heat all the time, every second no matter what I'm doing, no matter where I am. And at night, the warm impulses increase with higher temperature heat. I feel so warm - it's so warm. I'm so warm at night I can actually see by body glowing fire-orange red! And I know **TRILLIONS OF CANCER CELLS ARE BEING KILLED** *by all this toasty warm glowing heat.*

Every time I breathe-in, the air going into my body turns fire-orange red - **KILLING TRILLIONS OF CANCER CELLS** *and heats up my body from the inside - it warms-up my blood which in turn warms-up every part of my body especially my feet, toes, hands and fingers! When I breathe-out, cold air and* **CANCEROUS TOXINS** *leave my body. When I breathe-in and hold my breath the fire-orange red air goes from warm too HOT to give my body extra HOT heat. My body is so extra warm when I do this that I can see my body glowing even during daylight hours!*

I am so warm that I want to take-off my jacket but I'll keep it on. I feel so warm, I glow like a fire fly and I know **MY ENTIRE BODY IS BEING CLEANSED COMPLETELY FROM CANCER!** *I feel so warm I glow like a florescent lamp. I feel so warm that any rain drops that do hit my clothes, just turn into vapor and evaporate. "*

Got the idea? You can make your own visualizations that touch the subconscious mind - the subconscious mind which is more powerful than you can imagine! Before we leave the subject of color, let me give you a true example how color can manipulate the mind.

The following is a direct quote from one of my other Survival Books found at **www.survivalexpertbooks.com** – *"375+ International Prisoner Survival Tricks And More!"*

Prisoner Pink: Sheriff Joe Arpaio out of Phoenix, Arizona wanted to change the attitude of the prisoners in his jail, so when it came time to repainting the jail, he had all the prisoner cells painted pink. Why? After doing his research, he found that the color pink (not hot pink) is supposed to have a calming effect. So he thought, why not have the prisoners see pink where ever they look, thus calming them down - thus decreasing prison violence. This calming effect will lower prisoner violence against other prisoners and prison guards. This simply has a little safer environment for everyone. And yes colors do have Mind-Over-Matter effect - IF YOU BELIEVE!!!!!

Note: This segment should tell you that Color Therapy does work.

Corn Can Heal: The Anasazi grew crops and it was a most important food for their survival. And I told you about this indestructible food in the July 2001 AASN. Why is the corn such a good food? Well besides its cultivility (is this a word?) in the unforgiving desert environment, corn provides what the body needs. Here's a quote from the Gettysburg Program:

"A cup of cooked corn furnishes only 178 calories while a cup of creamed style corn furnishes 210 calories. Corn is low in sodium and low in fat. A **high energy food, corn is full of iron, zinc, niacin and rich in potassium as well as a great source of fiber.** Most people think of corn as a vegetable, so I put it in with the vegetable section. Corn is really a grain. Corn has been noted to have the healing properties of **controlling high blood pressure, fight heart disease, lowers cholesterol, lowers risk of cancer** due to its high fiber content and helps prevent dental cavities. Corn also contains the protease inhibitor chemicals that are cancer suppressors.

A worldwide study reported in 1981 by Pelayo Correa of the Louisiana State University Medical Center, noted a strong correlation between **low death rates from breast, colon and prostate cancer and heart disease and increased per capita consumption of sweet corn as well as beans and rice!**

Another survey of 47 countries found that areas where people consumed starch in corn rather than wheat or rice had **lower rates of dental cavities!**

According to Dr. Virgil Brown of Mount Sinai School of Medicine in New York; the Tarahumara Indians of Mexico eat corn and beans and not much else. **High blood cholesterol and cardiovascular heart disease are almost non-existent** among the Tarahumara Indians!"

WARNING: According to studies by Kenneth Carroll at the University of Western Ontario, corn oil was noted to cause cancer in lab animals. Corn oil was noted to lower immunity in mice."

Central & South American 03 Common Foods: I've eaten meals throughout Central and South America. I've eaten meals in restaurants, mess halls in military garrisons and even in the middle of nowhere in the dense humid jungles.

Many of these meals have 01, 02 or all these food ingredients in the main meal or complimenting the main meal no matter if it's a breakfast meal, lunch meal or dinner meal.

These 03 tasty food ingredients are:
- Beans
- Corn (kernel)
- Rice.

Add any or all these 03 food ingredients to your meals and you'll find you have a tastier and fuller meal. But for this recipe, we'll make a **full meal** (this meal will fill you up – it surely feels me up - MMMMmmmmmmm) using all three ingredients and we'll add toasted tortillas. OK, let's get started.

Ingredients: Stove, frying pan with cover, spoon, timer, 01 cup of Armour Chili With Beans Original (see *Chili With Beans Taste Test (06)*), 01 cup of already cooked white rice, 05 tablespoons of butter or margarine, 01 cup of sweet corn (Green Giant Whole Kernel Sweet Corn) salt & pepper and at least 07 tortillas. Add cold drink.

Step 01:   Add 02 tablespoons of butter or margarine into the frying pan and turn the heat on LOW. Let the butter or margarine melt till you go on to the next step.

Step 02:   Add the cup of beans in one separate section of the frying pan.

Step 03:   Add the white rice in a heap in another separate section of the frying pan and place the tablespoon of butter or margarine on top of the rice.

Step 04:   Add the corn between the beans and the rice in the frying pan and place the tablespoon of butter or margarine on top of the corn. The melted tablespoons of butter will melt and steam, thus aid in the heating, cooking process and taste for all 03 main ingredients.

Step 05:   With the burner on LOW and cover the frying pan. Set the timer to 50-minutes.

Step 06:   Periodically check the cooking process. If you want, stir or rotate the beans, rice and corn within their own section of the frying pan (Do Not mix the ingredients with each other). However, I have found there is no need to rotate or stir any of the ingredients. Just leave it alone. It will all heat-up and cook-up on its own.

Step 07: At approximately 50-minutes, when the beans, rice and corn are 'sizzling' and cooked to your liking, remover the frying pan from the burner to a cold burner.

Step 08: Immediately add the tortilla to the burner and turn the burner on MEDIUM HIGH.

Step 09: After 10-seconds or less, CAREFULLY CAREFULLY grab the tortilla on its very edge WITHOUT WITHOUT touching the burner and turn it over.

Step 10: Repeat this process till the tortilla is HOT and toasted on both sides. Turn OFF the burner.

Step 11: Sprinkle on some salt & pepper. Notice that there is no eating bowl in the recipe. Eat this hot meal right out of the frying pan. Use the tortilla (tear off sections) to scoop-up each of the tasty ingredients (or use a spoon).

To eat this meal with a tortilla, you'll need at least 07 toasted tortillas. ENJOY with your cold drink.

1st Note: If you want instead of using 01 cup of corn and 01 cup of beans for this recipe, use the entire can of corn and beans.

2nd Note: This is one of my favorite meals. I did add my own spices to this meal. See *Laydon's Super Spice Combo For Taste And Healing*.

With this meal you can spoon or fork some hot rice, chili bean or corn separately or you can do a double or triple combination with it using a fork, spoon or section of toasted tortilla - MMMmmmmmm!!

Indestructible Food You Gotta Have In Your Backpack:
Here's an indestructible food you gotta have in your backpack for emergency food. It's corn! Yes corn! Corn is not only indestructible, it provides those carbohydrates needed for energy and it will give you that filled-up feeling so you won't feel hungry! Let me give you some background information to appreciate this valuable food source.

It's Alive!

Those hard kernels of corn might look like it's dead on the outside but on the inside it's alive! That outer shell protects the seed on the inside. It does such a good job to protect it that if it stays dry it will last years and years and years!

As a matter of fact, scientist found old popcorn kernels at Bat Cave, New Mexico that were approximately 2,000 years old! And did this 2,000-year old popcorn still pop? It sure did! An indestructible food source! Heck, you can put popcorn kernels in your bigger survival kits and you'll never have to mess with it again till you need it for emergency food!

Inside each kernel of corn is a seed along with a minute portion of water. When heat is applied to the kernel the water heats, turns to vapor, the vapor expands and swells the kernel. The hot steam escapes and air rushes in forming puffy popped corn.

But to grow the corn, simple water will slowly dissolve and break away the hard outer shell. But in your survival situation you don't have time (several months) to grow corn and wait to harvest it. You want food now. So your best bet is popcorn. All it takes is some heat to pop it.

A 02-pound bag of popcorn will provide plenty of FILLING emergency food for many days! So pack a 02-pound bag of popcorn in an airtight & water-proof container for your bigger survival kits (car, boat, snowmobile, plane, truck, house, cabin,...) and 1/2-pound bag in your backpack so you're ready Anytime Anywhere!

Note: There are many different types of corn. Some corn pops and some doesn't. Insure you pack regular popping popcorn. Yes they come in different size kernels for different sizes of puffy popcorn! I always purchase white and yellow popcorn. Both are delicious.

Delicious Treat For Immediate Energy: You might be feeling weak so I thought I'd add this segment in here. I was doing some research on Chronic Fatigue Syndrome and came across a remedy for it. I was feeling slow and weak and gave it a try. Guess what happened?

It worked! May be it was all in my head, but who cares it worked anyway. The remedy is cocoa.

Meaning I bought some chocolate candy to eat. But not any chocolate – <u>it has to be dark chocolate</u>. I went and bought a whole bag of bite size dark chocolate candies and put them in the freezer (taste even better frozen). Hershey offers a few candies. Look for the words *"Special Dark."*

Coue's Auto-Suggestion: Frenchman Emile Coue is the Father of Autosuggestion. Autosuggestion is the art and belief that stating aimed positive affirmations several times a day (morning and night) towards that affliction (example), autosuggestions will remedy that affliction. In 1857, Coue discovered the power of the mind when one of his patients was cured by his own mind and not the medicine he was given which turned out to be a placebo.

Coue studied with A.A. Liebeault who was a hypnotist. Liebeault helped cure patients of their afflictions via hypnosis. Coue concluded that the real healing is within the patient (their mind). He then conducted *"intensive research"* to find how a way to trigger the patient's own healing ability.

He came up with what is now known as Autosuggestion. Coue simply told his patients to say one phrase several times a day - preferably after they wake-up in the morning and before they go to sleep because the conscious mind is more receptive to suggestion at these times.

Coue's patients were given several autosuggestions but the most popular one was *"Every day in every way I am getting better and better."*

Coue died in 1926 but his work didn't die with him. Autosuggestion is practiced worldwide and you just did it yourself - OK, one more time - *"Every day in every way I am getting better and better."*

DETOX DETOX DETOX: I'm no highly educated doctor nor a qualified nurse but I do know when it comes to getting your body to heal-up and fight-off all kinds of maladies in the first place is you gotta DETOX DETOX DETOX your body so your IMMUNE SYSTEM can more readily do its job to keep you vibrantly healthy.

So here's a list of DETOXES in this Survival Book that you gotta take a re-look at:

- Amazing Gua Sha Detox
- Clean Yourself Up From The Inside With Amazing Chelation Therapy
- Fasting Kills Cancer
- Fourteen Healing Oils You Can't Live Without (Castor Oil)
- More Healing Black Dirt
- The Five Deadly Whites
- The Mother Of All Antioxidants
- Tumeric

Devil's Claw: The Khoison peoples of the Kalahari Desert have used the roots of the Devil's Claw for centuries. Devil's Claw is a Kalahari desert plant.

It can be identified by its red flowers, wild spinach looking leaves, and carrot-looking roots - tubers. Devil's Claw has been used by native Africans for centuries to remedy pain and other maladies. In the early 1900s, it was introduced to Europe. Devil's Claw may work where other medicines have failed. Devil's Claw is used to remedy:

- Allergies
- Appetite Restoration
- Arthritis Pain
- Arthritis Stiffness
- Back Pain
- Chronic Pain
- Chronic Stomach Problems
- Digestive Problems
- Fever
- Headaches
- Heartburn
- Improves Joint Flexibility
- Inflammation Reduction
- Joint Pain
- Muscle Aches & Pains
- Muscle Spasms
- Neck Pain
- Pregnancy Complications
- Relieves Osteoarthritis
- Skin Boils
- Skin Problems
- Skin Sores
- Skin Ulcers
- Stomach Pain

According to nutritional expert Earl Mindell, R.Ph., Ph.D. *"...it's a uniquely powerful pain reliever, able to shut down some of the most stubborn aches and pains known..."*

Some of the Devil's Claw healing ingredients may be due to its iridoid glycosides, harposides,... Devil's Claw is made in capsule form, tablets, liquid extracts, topical ointments, and tea (infused). Devil's Claw can be found at your local healthfood store.

Diabetes Risk Reducer: Diabetes is striking down more people than ever before. According to a study, people with Type 2 Diabetes dropped their blood sugar levels by 13%. How?

They soaked in a hot tub of 102-degrees F. for 30-minutes, 06-days a week for 03-weeks. This hot soaking increases blood circulation - thus dropping blood sugar levels.

Doctor Vernon's Diabetes Remedy: Doctor Vernon out of Lawrence, Kansas - USA, prescribes a diabetes remedy to his patients the old fashion way. *"People walk into her office afflicted with Type 2 Diabetes and, by every objective medical measurement, walk out cured."*

Dr. Vernon states: *"My first line of treatment is to have patients remove carbohydrates from their diets. This is often all it takes to REVERSE their symptoms, so that they NO LONGER REQUIRE MEDICATION."*

"I believe in in addressing the cause, not the symptoms" she says. *"That's why I first eliminate the foods that raise blood sugar. It's only logical."*

In 2003, researchers at Duke University set out to test Dr. Vernon's findings. The 16-week study found that 17 out of the 21 participants significantly reduced their medication or discontinued it all together.

Dr. Vernon is definitely on the right track. Check this out –

A study of Greenland's Eskimos (Inuit) in which prior to the 1980s, they had the **LOWEST PREVALENCE OF HEART DISEASE AND DIABETES ON THE ENTIRE PLANET. A 25-year study found that one 01, only 01, only 01 out of 1,800 Eskimos monitored developed diabetes. Again, that's just 01 out of 1,800!!** What's their secret? A diet entirely of fat and protein with <u>only 03% of it from carbohydrates</u>. See *Eskimo Diabetes Cure*.

Drinking Pure Water Fights Cancer: According to a located at Seattle, Washington, women who drank at least 04 glasses of water each day <u>reduced their chance of killer colon cancer by 50%</u>! Why does it work?

According to Ann Shattuck, an epidemiologist, hydration of water turns the intestinal tract including the colon into a *"express train"* that eliminates possible carcinogens (cancer-causing bad guys) that could turn into cancer if they had a chance to hang around. It may also have the same effect on the urinary tract, the bladder, the kidneys, ureter,...

According to another research at the Cancer Research Center located in Hawaii, women who drank the most tap water (I bet it was pure water compared to contaminated water found within the continental US), <u>had an 80% less chance of developing bladder cancer</u>. According to Lynne Wilkens: *"The more they drank, the higher the reduction of risk."*

According to British researchers, <u>women *"water drinkers"* had a smaller risk of breast cancer than those women who didn't drink plenty of water</u>.

Emergency First-Aid For A Heart Attack Victim, 1st:
The following is CPR (Cardiopulmonary Resuscitation) for the **UNTRAINED**.

- Apply uninterrupted chest compressions of 100 to 120 compressions per minute till paramedics arrive on the scene.

Emergency First-Aid For A Heart Attack Victim, 2nd:
The following is a herbal remedy for a victim of a heart attack. Here are 02 quotes worthy of your attention:

"If you master one herb in your life, master cayenne pepper. It is more powerful than any other herb."
Dr. Richard Schulze

"In 35 years of practice, and working with the people, and teaching, I have never on house calls lost one heart attack patient, and the reason is, whenever I go in, if they are still breathing, I pour down them a cup of cayenne tea: a teaspoon of cayenne in a cup of hot water, and within minutes they are up and around."

Dr. John R. Christopher

For proof of the healing effectiveness cayenne pepper, please read / re-read:

- Capsicum (cayenne)
- Laydon's Healing Spice Concoction
- Richard Quinn's Heart Disease Cure

Eskimo Diabetes Cure: The Yup'ik Eskimos in Alaska eat 20-times more Omega-3 fats from the fish they eat than Americans in the lower 48 states. A high intake of Omega-3 fats suggest this high intake may **PREVENT obesity-related chronic diseases like diabetes** and heart disease.

A study of Greenland's Eskimos (Inuit) in which prior to the 1980s, they had the **LOWEST PREVALENCE (widespread) OF HEART DISEASE AND DIABETES ON THE ENTIRE PLANET. A 25-year study found that one (01), only 01, only 01 out of 1,800 Eskimos monitored developed diabetes. Again, that's 01 out of 1,800 Eskimos!!** What the heck is going on? What the heck is their secret? Their secret is a diet entirely of fat and protein with <u>only 03% of it from carbohydrates</u>. You have to re-read *Doctor Vernon's Diabetes Remedy*.

Exercise Mind-Over-Matter Trick: Need to exercise but just can't get out of bed? Then here's a neat Mind-Over-Matter application worthy of your attention. I strongly believe in Mind-Over-Matter applications because they have happened to me and you can read about em' in one of my books - *"72+ Fantastic Mind-Over-Matter Applications You Have To Know And More!"* found at   **www.survivalexpertbooks.com**

And like I always said, *"If you don't believe ain't nuthin' gonna happen!"* Here's a Mind-Over-Matter application that's backed-up by a wise researcher and scientific proof!

First of all, your conscious mind knows the difference between what is real life and what is fantasy. But your subconscious doesn't know the difference. That's why many Mind-Over-Matter applications tap into the subconscious so the user does the impossible.

According to Dave Smith, Ph.D., a sports psychologist at Chester College, England *"We found that the parts of the brain that control movement are stimulated by thinking about movement."*

And muscle increases the metabolism which burns calories - fat even when you sleep.

"To a certain extent, the mind (subconscious mind) can't tell the difference between really doing something and imagining it. You need to imagine that you are actually doing something athletic."

Dave Smith, Ph.D., says you don't have to sweat you need to CONCENTRATE. *"Close your eyes and imagine how you'd move your body, what it would feel like."*

Dr. Smith states **just 05 concentrated minutes a day should do the trick.** That 05-minutes a day translates into 22-pounds a year! Want proof?

Dr. Smith did a study at Manchester Metropolitan University using 03 groups of people. The 1st group concentrated on muscle contractions 20-times a day for a whole month. The 2nd group actually did the real exercise.

Dr. Smith found that the 2nd group that did the actual exercise, increased their strength by 33%.
The 1st group that imagined the muscle contractions increased their strength by 16%! The 3rd group that did nothing increased their strength by 0%.

Now who can use this Mind-Over-Matter application? YOU can! And YOU can do it just about anywhere (except driving or activities that endanger your life or other lives). Try doing it before you go to sleep at night. So try it, **BELIEVE IT,** YOU HAVE TO BELIEVE IT WORKS! Your mind is an AMAZING MACHINE no computer can match! See *Multiple Healing Wonders Of Rebound Exercise.*

Famous Willard Water: In November of 1980, **CBS' 60 Minutes** was sent to Rapid City, South Dakota, to do a feature called *"Doc's Wonder Water."* The CBS' 60 Minutes investigative team was sent to expose a fraud.

What they found was an amazing true story about a newly invented form of water which was actually producing what could only be called miraculous results! Catalyst Water has since been improved since 1980 and is made in an FDA-approved facility using the latest in state-of-the-art mixing, filling and processing equipment.

Water is the most important biological factor sustaining living organisms. Water molecules improve and speed up cell movement, nutrients moving into and out of living organisms cells.

Catalyst water is pure ordinary water which has been treated with a catalyst. The catalyst appears to change the molecular structure of the water, making the molecules smaller.

When this happens, the water becomes more penetrable, and anything dissolved in the water like beneficial nutrients from food, minerals and Vitamins is more readily absorbed into our bodies. Smaller water molecules are able to penetrate the cell walls at a greater rate and carry beneficial nutrients to where it needs to be.

The bio-enhanced water is also unique with a pH (percentage of hydrogen) of 12 which means bacteria can not live in a high pH.

The inventor also states that his "water" also contains small amounts of several harmless ingredients such as liquid road salt, sodium silicate, magnesium sulfate and sulfated castor oil.

Catalyst Water was invented by Dr. John Wesley Willard (Doc). Also known as "Bio-Enhanced" or "Catalyst-Enhanced" Water. Catalyst Water is non-toxic, non-carcinogenic and has been used for over 20 years without anyone having any adverse reaction or adverse effects from it!

Catalyst Water can be used internally and externally. Below is a list of recorded testimonial benefits of the REAL Willard Water!

Human Effects!

- Aches Reduced
- Alertness
- Antioxidant
- Arthritis
- Back Problems
- Bronchitis
- Calming Effect
- Circulation (feet & hands)
- Colds (fewer)
- Complexion Color
- Constipation
- Energy
- Food Absorption
- Free Radical Scavenger
- Hair Improvement
- Happier
- Healing (quicker)
- Hemorrhoids
- Sutures (fast healing - spray with WW)
- Memory Improvement
- Nail Improvement
- Nutrient Absorption
- Nutritional Supplements Work Better
- Pain Reduced
- Reduced Swelling
- Skin Rashes
- Sleep Improvement
- Stress Reducer
- Toxin & Waste Elimination

Note: Besides drinking WW, some people sprayed the malady directly with WW or soaked in a bathtub treated with WW. And what about critters? If WW worked for humans why not critters? Here are some testimonial results from happy pet owners.

Animal Effects!

- Anti-social
- Arthritis
- Calming Effect
- Longevity
- Overall Health
- Performance (greyhounds)

My Results!

Folks for this research (July - August 2001) I purchased an 08-ounce bottle of *The Real Willard Water!* I purchased the darker color of Willard Water because it had a bunch of additional minerals that the clear Willard Water doesn't have. Anyway, the health results do sneak up on you. But two that stood out immediately are ENERGY and SLEEP IMPROVEMENT.

I since stopped taking any Willard Water and no doubt know there's a degradation of energy and sleep. As you read this, I'm back on Willard Water, but instead of buying the small bottle, you get a MUCH BETTER DEAL when you buy the bigger bottles which last a lot longer! You just add 1-ounce of concentrated Willard Water to a gallon of pure water and you got a **GALLON OF WILLARD WATER!**

WARNING: In the Gettysburg Program, I gave you a FAKE catalyst water POC - I'm sorry, I got fooled too. Go to the POC Section and get a POC for the AUTHENTIC WILLARD WATER! Don't believe a word of this segment. Call right now and they'll send you a **FREE** multi-page brochure on this amazing special water that helps your body heal!

Follow the recommended dosage and instructions from the label and as per your doctor's instructions.

Fasting Kills Cancer: CANCER LOVES SUGAR. CANCER LOVES SUGAR. CANCER LOVES SUGAR. CANCER LOVES SUGAR. CANCER LOVES SUGAR. CANCER LOVES SUGAR. CANCER LOVES SUGAR. CANCER LOVES SUGAR. Why? **Cancer has 'sugar receptors.'** It loves and eats sugar so it can grow.

OK, did I make my point? You have to STOP eating *The Five Deadly Whites* and start fasting. STOP eating ALL foods that have any sugar. Go on a very restrictive diet so to DETOX your body and at the same time you're STARVING the cancer of food it needs to live and grow.

Note: When my Momma was dying from cancer, the powers to be (her doctors) had her drinking these cans of delicious milkshake-like drinks. They really tasted good but they were LOADED LOADED LOADED with SUGAR! Back then, I had no idea that CANCER LOVES SUGAR. Now I do and so do you! See *The Five Deadly Whites*. Also see the following YouTube videos annotated in the POC Section:

- Cancer Cure – Baking Soda And Molasses

- Cancer Disappears With Water Fasting - Dr. Alan Goldhamer
- Fasting Kills Cancer
- Water Fasting Kills Cancer Cells

Fourteen Healing Oils You Can't Live Without:
"Fourteen Healing Oils You Can't Live Without And More" gives you fourteen oils that have international history and international healing benefits. Let me briefly tell you about each healing oil.

Let's start with Shark Liver Oil.

<u>Shark Liver Oil</u> has been used for centuries and has now drawn the attention of scientist, doctors, and health enthusiast all around the world.

<u>Olive Oil</u> is used by Mediterranean people who have been noted to develop far less heart disease than Americans.

<u>Omega-3 Fatty Acids</u> have successfully blocked both migraine headaches and kidney disease.

<u>Castor Oil</u> is a POTENT CLEANSER - DETOXIFIER. Flaxseed Oil and low-fat cottage cheese was prescribed by Dr. Johanna Budwig to seriously ill cancer patients. Over a period of approximately 90 days, tumors gradually receded.

Oil of Oregano's wide and long resume of healings throughout history to the present day are very impressive. Without any assistance from other natural remedies or synthetic drugs, oregano kills fungus or blocks its growth. Oil of Oregano also attacks and outright destroys antibiotic-resistant super-germs, bacteria, molds, parasites, viruses, yeast,...

Clove Oil goes after the bad guys (germicide, bactericide,…). It STOPPED my non-stop pounding toothache pain within a couple minutes.

Wheat Germ Oil is a valuable dietary supplement to men doing hard exercise, and it has possible application to competitive sports. It provides something that enables men to bear hard stress and continue to do hard labor without deteriorating.

Coconut Oil is rich in what is called lauric acid which is found in Mother's milk. Lauric acid has anti-bacteria, anti-fungal, and anti-viral agents. The super healthy fresh coconut oil and fresh white meat have a laundry list of super healthy benefits.

Panaseeda Oil - I read about a German - a 1996 Olympian named Andreas Wecker who won a Gold Medal on the High Bar and won other Olympic Medals. An athlete in phenomenal shape who years later (early 2000s), his health declined in the worst way. In 2005 his health declined so much he weighed-in at a sickly 84 pounds.

Andreas Wecker was diagnosed with chronic sickness called Crohn's disease (inflammatory bowel disease). Close to death, Andreas Wecker turned to an alternative treatment where every conventional method failed. He turned to what is now called Panaseeda Oil.

Fish Oil brought dramatic relief to inflammation and stiff joints caused by rheumatoid arthritis. Migraines generally eased up in about 60 percent of those who took fish oil capsules for six weeks.

Tea Tree Oil is composed of 98 compounds and 06 oil compositions. Tea Tree Oil has antifungal properties, antimicrobial properties, antiseptic properties, and inflammatory properties.

Turpentine Oil - this is no snake oil. Instead of giving you a good write-up on this unknown healer, I decided to give you a 03-part video so you can get the healing wonders straight from the horse's mouth!

Krill Oil also provides canthaxanthin, a potent anti-oxidant. The anti-oxidant potency of krill oil compared to fish oil in terms of ORAC (Oxygen Radical Absorptance Capacity) values it was found to be 48 times more potent than fish oil.

Flax Seed Oil. Seriously ill cancer patients were treated with flax seed oil and low-fat cottage cheese by Dr. Johanna Budwig. Over a period of approximately 90 days, tumors gradually receded.

Symptoms of anemia, cancer, diabetes and liver dysfunction were completely alleviated!

Plus, a **SECRET** BONUS HEALER in this book. All this healthy and beneficial information and MUCH MORE in this book.

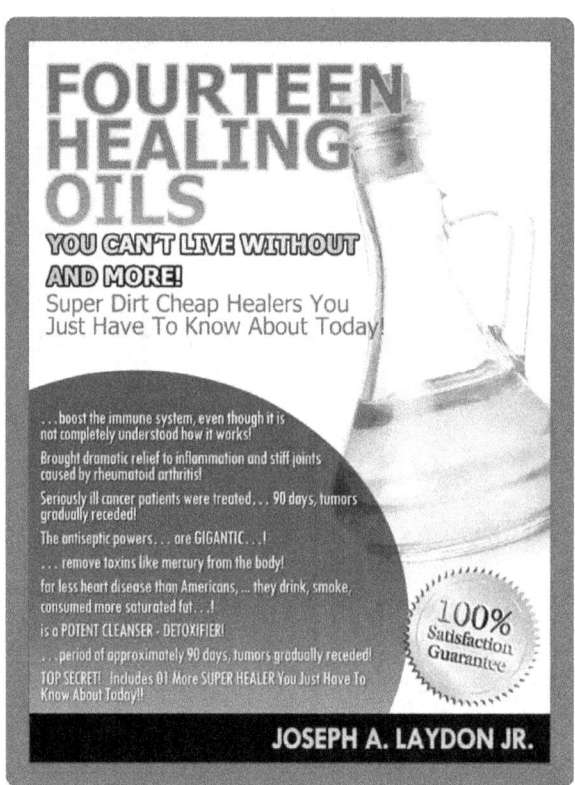

Simply go to **www.amazon.com** and type-in the title to get the complete 149-page book.

Gamma Linolenic Acid (GLA): GLA is a regulator of T-lymphocyte function in your body. GLA can be made from linolenic acid which is found in vegetable oils as long as you're not deficient in magnesium and Vitamins A, B3, B6, C, and zinc (conversion may be blocked).

Pre-formed sources of GLA are black currant seed oil, borage oil, and evening primrose oil.

Many diabetics may be LOW in essential fatty acids due to the Standard American Diet which is lacking in essential fatty acids as well as many vital nutrients (Vitamins and micronutrients).

According to a 1993 study in England in which 111 diabetic participants consumed 480mg of GLA on a daily basis for one year; <u>**improvements were noted "in several parameters" especially neuropathy. This micronutrient may help ameliorate a diabetic condition!**</u>

YOU MUST SEE *Biotin*, *Chromium Picolinate*, *Vanadyl Sulfate* as well as *Gymnema Sylvestre* in this book.

WARNING: Hydrogenated vegetable oils, margarine, or a high-fat diet may also inhibit the conversion to GLA!

Follow the recommended dosage and instructions from the label and as per your doctor's instructions.

Graviola: *"There are approximately 300,000 types of plants that grow on the earth's surface, in salt water and in fresh water. Of these 300,000 plants on Earth, 120,000 varieties are edible."*

And I believe of all these 300,000+ plants both non-edible and edible, some have super healing ingredients to fight the most deadliest diseases known to man and diseases that are hitting us now (SARS), and diseases of the future. Yes, even NBC (nuclear, biological, chemical) threats.

One such healing wonder plant is from the beautiful greenish, thick and unforgiving Amazon Rainforest, the plant is called *Graviola*. Savvy Amazon Indians used *Graviola* for arthritis, boils, diarrhea neuralgia, dysentery, flu, hypertension, insomnia, malaria, muscle spasm, rashes, rheumatism, ringworm, scurvy, ulcers,... Back in the early 1990s, a drug company _____, thought *Graviola* might be a potential money-maker.

What they found was that *Graviola* was a stalking predator to 12 different types of cancer. It tracked down and went after 12 different types of cancer cells WITHOUT harming any other cells around the sickly deadly cancer cells. They found that *Graviola* was estimated to be **10,000-times more potent** than expensive top of the line chemotherapy drugs! And using *Graviola*, there was no hair-loss, nausea, weight-loss, immune system damage,... that's associated with chemotherapy treatment.

The drug company knew they couldn't patent *Graviola*, so they attempted to synthesize it. Their R & D went on for several years but all their attempts failed so they kept *Graviola* to themselves. Why? Cause *Graviola* could actually hurt their business. *Graviola* could outperform cancer drugs they were currently selling to millions of cancer patients. Luckily for us, an insider went public on *Graviola*.

Where can you find more information on *Graviola*? It's from *Health Sciences Institute* (keep reading). And there are **many more supplements** that are worthy of your attention, too many to annotate in this segment, so you have to get on *Health Sciences Institute's* mailing list today. See *Graviola And How It Can Heal The Cancer* in the POC Section.

Healing And Performance Wonders You're Not Supposed To Know About: You ever hear those stories about those ingenious inventors making automobiles so fuel-efficient that the big car companies buy their invention(s) and permanently shut-up the inventors by putting millions of dollars in their pockets!! Yes this is a potential future write-up but I want you to know about natural *"healing wonders you're not supposed to know about"* and suppressed by drug companies cause they can't make a dime off them or will lose business if a natural remedy is found to be <u>more effective</u> than their current synthetic drugs. Healing and performance wonders that can't be patented, therefore not a money-maker. Plus, other healing and performance wonders you must know about.

Before I start, <u>**you must promise me to not believe a single word I'm telling you**</u> in this segment. Below is a POC to write them so to get on their mailing list today so you can get their **FREE** healing and performance information straight from the "horses mouth" - promise me - OK then! This segment's sole purpose is to get you to write the folks below and get on their mailing list today. OK then, let's start.

I've always said *"Mother Nature and all She possesses is trying to kill you dead 100 different ways. But at the same time She's also trying to help you out a 1,000 different ways!"* Whether you're 21 or 121, Mother Nature has plenty of plants on this Earth to feed you and heal you, and help prevent disease from the get go.

As I stated in Package 01 - Section 07 - Field-Expedient Plant Procurement: *"There are approximately 300,000 types of plants that grow on the earth's surface, in salt water and in fresh water. Of these 300,000 plants on Earth, 120,000 varieties are edible."*

69

And I believe of all these 300,000+ plants both non-edible and edible, some have super healing ingredients to fight the most deadliest diseases known to man and diseases that are hitting us now (SARS), and diseases of the future. Yes, even NBC (nuclear, biological, chemical) threats.

One such healing wonder plant is from the beautiful greenish, thick and unforgiving Amazon Rainforest, the plant is called *Graviola*. Savvy Amazon Indians used *Graviola* for arthritis, boils, diarrhea neuralgia, dysentery, flu, hypertension, insomnia, malaria, muscle spasm, rashes, rheumatism, ringworm, scurvy, ulcers,...

Back in the early 1990s, a drug company _____, thought *Graviola* might be a potential money-maker. What they found was that *Graviola* was a stalking predator to 12 different types of cancer.

It tracked down and went after 12 different types of cancer cells WITHOUT harming any other cells around the sickly deadly cancer cells. They found that *Graviola* was estimated to be **10,000-times more potent** than expensive top of the line chemotherapy drugs! And using *Graviola*, there was no hair-loss, nausea, weight-loss, immune system damage,... that's associated with chemotherapy treatment.

The drug company knew they couldn't patent *Graviola*, so they attempted to synthesize it. Their R&D went on for several years but all their attempts failed so they kept *Graviola* to themselves. Why?

Cause *Graviola* could actually hurt their business. *Graviola* could outperform cancer drugs they were currently selling to millions of cancer patients. Luckily for us, an insider went public on *Graviola*.

Where can you find more information on *Graviola*? It's from *Health Sciences Institute* (keep reading). And there are **many more supplements** that are worthy of your attention, too many to annotate in this segment, so you have to get on *Health Sciences Institute's* mailing list today.

IMPORTANT NOTE: See this AASN (Acupressure, Bubblegum, Chocolate, Cinnamon, Devil's Claw, Healing Elk Antlers, Homeostatic Soil Organisms - HSOs, Indian Gator-Aid, Indium, Stress Busters, Whey,...), other AASNs, Special Reports, and the Gettysburg Program for many more healing and performance wonders! See 1999-2004 A-Z Index now!

Heath Sciences Institute--------------------------
number unavailable
Heath Sciences Institute, P.O. Box 925, Frederick, MD 21705-9913.

Healing Black Dirt: Find some rich black dirt and you may find some healing dirt that may remedy several maladies.

And now there's evidence that rich black dirt may contain a specific healing bacterial ingredient. There's good bacteria and bad bacteria and rich black dirt may contain good bacteria called homeostatic soil organisms (HSOs).

HSOs when in the human body, destroy dangerous organisms that are bad for our health like molds, parasites, yeast, and other microorganisms that interfere with proper digestion and absorption of food.

Millions and millions of North Americans are sickly because their HSOs intake is deficient. According to Jordan Rubin, N.D. *"...soils have been depleted of HSOs, and out intake has dropped."*

Research indicates that as many as 92% of people suffering from many gastrointestinal problems from indigestion to irritable bowel syndrome could find relief in 04-months from taking HSOs. According to Paul Goldberg, D.C. *"HSOs help crowd out the bad organisms that prevent proper digestion and trigger pain."*

And HSOs may offer some fighting help when it comes to preventing arthritis. According to gastroenterologist Joseph Brasco, M.D., coauthor of *Restoring Your Digestive Health* - *"Research shows that the more HSOs people eat, the lower their risk of ever developing arthritis."*

And HSOs may offer some help to remedy asthma and allergies. According to the National Institute of Allergy and Infectious Diseases, 35 million Americans are afflicted with allergies or asthma. According to Paul Goldberg, *"...when patients take 04 to 18 HSO caplets daily for 04 months, their asthma and allergy symptoms are reduced by 70%. When immune cells are regularly exposed to healthy HSOs, they learn to stop overreacting to dust, animal dander, pollen, and other harmless particles in the environment. That means less lung, airway, and sinus inflammation."*

HSOs are known to help prevent and or remedy:
- Asthma
- Constipation
- Food Allergies
- Heartburn
- Indigestion

- Irritable Bowel Syndrome
- Joint Stiffness
- Pain
- Rheumatoid Arthritis

No you don't have to go look for and eat rich black dirt to get your intake of healthy HSOs. HSOs can be found at local healthfood stores. And see the *Vitamin Shoppe* in the POC Section.

Follow the recommended dosage and instructions from the label and as per your doctor's instructions.

More Healing Black Dirt: We may have come from the oceans millions of years ago, but we humans may be solidly connected to the Earth's soil. Microbes found in the soil called Homeostatic Soil Organisms (HSOs - beneficial bacteria, good bacteria) are proving to be the super healers for the human body and probably all sorts of animal critters too.

According to Jo Handelsman, a professor of plant pathology at the University of Wisconsin, *"Unknown organisms make up 99.9% of all microbes in the soil."* About 01 gram of soil (equal to a packet of sugar), may contain as many as 10,000 unknown species.

Answers to curing cancers, heart disease, degenerative diseases, auto-immune diseases, obesity,... may be right under our feet - found in healthy soil. With the earth's soil depleted of nutrients like HSOs, it's no wonder that more than 85% of all Americans (author's estimate) are sickly, and dying.

But to prove the efficacy of HSOs where everything else has failed, let me relate a true life-saving story, a testimonial for HSOs. Before we start let me give a direct quote from the Gettysburg Program about a sickly and deadly disease - Crohn's Disease.

** (Direct quote from the Gettysburg Program): *"Crohn's disease is a chronic granulomatous inflammatory disease of unknown etiology, involving any part of the gastrointestinal tract from the mouth to the anus, but commonly involving the terminal ileum (the distal portion of the small intestine extending from the jejunum to the cecum), with scarring and thickening of the bowel wall. It frequently leads to intestinal obstruction and fistula (an abnormal passage) and abscess formation (a localized collection of pus caused by suppuration buried in tissues, organs or confined spaces) and has a high rate of recurrence after treatment. And colitis is inflammation of the bowel."*

In 1994, super-healthy 19-year old, 6'1" Jordan Rubin was a scholarship student at Florida State University who was suddenly stricken with Crohn's colitis. Once the disease was diagnosed, it was treated with massive doses of antibiotics (intravenous and oral). These massive doses of antibiotics only worsened his sickly condition.

Jordan was desperately fighting for his life. His weight went from a healthy 180-pounds to a sickly 104-pounds. Jordan and his family sought help from more than 70 health professionals around the world. He even consumed more than 300 nutritional supplements but nothing detoured his slow path to a sickly death. Jordan was finally sent home in a wheelchair to die.

Finally, in 1996, Jordan discovered a new supplement that contained HSOs. Taking HSOs complimented with a healthy diet, in 04-months, Jordan's health took a 180-degree turn for the better. With the HSO supplements, his body began to heal itself.

In only 04-months, he regained his healthy weight and did what 30 health professionals and 300 supplements couldn't do - he beat the sickly and deadly Crohn's colitis.

Today Jordan is as healthy as ever and weighs in at a healthy 195-pounds. Jordan didn't stop there though, he wrote a book about his life-threatening ordeal and his impressive recovery called *Patient Heal Thyself*.

How did these HSO help save Jordan's life? HSOs are noted to provide:

a) **Alpha-interferon**: Alpha-interferon is potent immune system enhancer and potent virus inhibitor. HSO's help promote the production of more natural alpha-interferons.

b) **Antigens**: Aid in the production of proteins that act as antigens that boost the immune system to manufacture antibodies to fight off disease.

c) **Fights Bad Guys**: Fights bacteria, fungi, parasites, pathological molds, and yeast.

d) **Hydrocarbons**: Hydrocarbons are better broken so to better break down food for its different nutritional values; thus allowing for better nutrition absorption.

e) **Intestines**: Flush out decay, debris, and waste from inside the intestines.

f) Lactoferrin: As a by-product, lactoferrin is manufactured which aids in retrieval of iron from foods. Lactoferrin is also found in women's breast milk and is a very powerful fighter of infection and disease. Lactoferrin now shows promise as a natural but very powerful cancer fighter.

g) Toxic Waste: Metabolize proteins to eliminate toxic waste from the body.

I (author) highly encourage you to go to your local library and get Jordan's book - *Patient Heal Thyself* so you're super healthy Anytime Anywhere! Now I know why I've never seen a sickly earth worm! Have you?

Ha ha ha!!! Seriously, for a quality HSO supplement see *Vitamin Shoppe* in the POC Section.

Most Important Note: The more I research about HSO's the more I like them good bacteria guys and the good they do for the body. But one fact I really like is that HSOs help **detoxify the body** so your body can help heal itself. By the time you read this, I'm already doing my own guinea pig tests (on myself) on an HSO product to see what it can do for me. So, again, I highly encourage you to look deeper into HSOs so Your More Healthy Anytime Anywhere!

Healing Elk Antlers: Now here's a supplement derived from the antlers of elk only found in northern Canada (Wapiti Elk - exact species unknown), to treat aching, painful, stiff, swelling,...
  • Ankles

- Backs
- Elbows
- Fingers
- Hips
- Knees
- Necks
- Shoulders
- Wrists,...!
-

It's being used to "repair... re-grow full, pain-free mobility to damaged joints, muscles, tendons, and cartilage.

What is this miracle wonder? It's marrow from the elk's antlers. According to Oxford University in England and Canadian Medical Schools: *"Elk Antler marrow is the fastest regenerating substance in all of nature."* The miracle substances found plentiful in this rare species of elk from northern Canada are anti-inflammatory prostaglandins and Type I & Type II regenerative collagen.

Now you don't have to go gnaw on some elk's antler while it's galloping through the dense forest of northern Canada; you can get a supplement called *FLEXAGENE*. And they're offering *FLEXAGENE* at a super low introductory price plus FREE gifts. See *Biogenetics, Inc.* in the POC Section now.

Note: Biogenetics Inc., also offers another supplement to relieve painful joints called *OPC Miracle Joint Complex*. OPC is similar to a supplement called *Pychnogenol*.

Healing Negative Ions: I'm telling you with the IRISAP Survival Program you have in front of you, you know more REAL wilderness survival than 99.9999% of folks walking this Earth! And did you notice when you're outdoor's you feel better - you feel good don't you! You know why? Cause it's because of negative ions! Negative ions are charged particles of oxygen.

According to Pierce J. Howard, Ph.D., author of *The Owner's Manual For The Brain*, multitudes of negative ions can be found near beaches, mountains and moving bodies of water. When negative ions are inhaled, they produce a chemical reaction within our bodies boosting serotonin levels that are instrumental in lifting our mood, making us feel much better.

Doctor Howard goes on to say *"The air at the beach contains negative ions, but in homes and offices, there may be only a few hundred - or even zero."* Getting a good helping of negative ions improves our health. Howard goes on to say *"The result is that our moods rise, our stress dissolves, we have more energy and we even sleep better at night."*

Ion researcher Michael Terman Ph.D., at Columbia University states, *"At the shore, it's the pounding of the surf on land that creates negative ions in the air. But thunderstorms do the same thing, by pounding the earth with heavy rains."* Terman goes on to say *"Negative ions seem to be most plentiful in humid environments. So if you expose yourself to humidity, you'll likely get an energizing and mood-lifting dose of negative ions."*

So if your not out in the wilderness, just step outside on your porch after a thunderstorm has <u>long passed</u> and get a good helping of negative ions - heck open up the windows to get the whole house full of negative ions!

So next time you're outdoors and are feeling blue, feeling down in the dumps, or a survivor in your group has a bad attitude, - instead of slapping that whacked-out survivor around or securing him 50-meters downwind next to your latrine, GO STATIC near a beach, moving water source, mountains,... or hunker down after a thunderstorm and collect some healing healthy negative ions and carry-on with the *8 Elements of Survival* (fire, water, shelter, first-aid, signal, food, weapons, and navigation).

Negative ions have been studied to have the following positive effects on the body:

- Improve one's energy
- Improve mood
- Fight depression
- Fight fatigue
- Reduce or eliminate stress
- Improve sleep

But what if I want negative ions in my home right now 24-hours a day? You can purchase a negative ion generator which are found at your local hardware stores.

Healing Orange Peels: First let me give you a quote from the Gettysburg Program concerning oranges, then I'll tell you about healing orange peels.

**Oranges: A medium orange furnishes only 62 calories, has virtually no sodium and hardly any fat, and is a great way to get your Vitamin C. The U.S. Department of Agriculture found that almost every milligram of Vitamin C in oranges do survive the transition from the orange grove to frozen orange juice concentrate.

Oranges lower the risk of some cancers, as well as effectively ***lowering blood cholesterol and fighting arterial plaque!***

A recent discovery by scientists found that an ingredient in orange peels may stop heartburn and remedy ulcers. Scientists stated the problem isn't because there is too much acid, it's because the body can't handle what acid is already there. Scientists found an ingredient in orange peels called DGL that boosts the body's natural defenses to handle acid. But there is an over-the-counter product that contains DGL that may help fight heartburn and ulcers, it's called *Pepstat 380* and available at most drug stores.

Note: As a kid, me and my friends weren't rich. When we ate oranges, we also ate the orange peels and they tasted real good! So next time you go outdoors and have an orange or two on you or find oranges in the wilderness, consider eating the orange peels to prevent or fight heartburn and ulcers.

Healing Pitch: No, I'm not talking about the pitch that comes from the processing of coal tar, wood tar or petroleum. I'm talking about readily available pitch, the sap that comes from coniferous trees like pine trees. Pitch ranges in color from a very light straw color to a deep dark brown color, and that sticky pitch has healing qualities. Pitch has been used long ago to treat gunshot wounds back in the Old West days and beyond. Why?

The ingredients in pitch are proven to offer anti-bacterial properties, anti-viral properties, infection-fighting properties, immune boosting properties,...

International studies and regular folks have used pitch
and pitch extracts to help remedy:

- Anti-Viral
- Burns (topical)
- Cuts (topical)
- Hemorrhoids (topical)
- Immune System Booster
- Nail Fungus
- Open Wounds (topical)
- Puncture Wounds (topical)
- Radiation Damage
- Ringworm (topical)
- Scabies (topical)
- Skin Abrasions (topical)
- Skin Ulcers (topical)
- Streptococcus Mutans (bacteria found in dental cavities)
- Warts (topical)

Now that you know the healing qualities of pitch, don't
get mad next time you go outdoor's, finding pine sap on
your gear, hands, clothes,... Collect some of it for
emergency fire-starting and emergency first-aid. But
if you want ready-to-go pitch products, here's a
company I listed several years ago.

The company is called NATR. You know what NATR stands
for - **N**ative **A**merican **T**ree **R**esin; and NATR offers some
amazing products that contain healing pitch (resin,
sap,...) from Douglas F896+5irs and Yellow Pines off
the California Pacific Coast. By the way, PAV contains
petroleum jelly. And you read about the healing and
survival uses of petroleum jelly - see *VPJ Inventor -
Robert Augustus Chesebrough*. And see NATR in the POC
Section.

MOST IMPORTANT NOTE: I myself (author) have been using

Healing Russian Arctic Weed (RAW): What the heck is Russian Arctic Weed (RAW)? RAW is now surfacing as a potent herb to aid in longevity and you can look towards many "vibrant & sharp as a whip" Russian farmers as proof. RAW has a history of being fed to Russians that really needed to be at their very best for the Mother Land - astronauts and Russian World Class Athletes.

a) Brain Power: A test group ate an extract of RAW and in 24-hours their test scores shot up an amazing **88%!** The control group that took a placebo scored 84% lower.

b) Anti-Depression: RAW is also noted to boost the "feel good" hormone - serotonin - by 30%, thus fighting depression.

c) Energy After-Burner: RAW is also noted to somehow boosts the energy levels. How it does this is unclear at the time of this writing.

f) Weight-Loss: As you just read if RAW could help boost energy levels it has to help you lose unwanted, unhealthy extra pounds.

A test group that took RAW supplements lost 20-pounds in a few months while the control group gained weight.

OK, I know what you're asking, where can you get more information on RAW? See *The Country Doctor's Big Bag Of Common Sense Cures* in the POC Section.

Healing Salve: Alexander Mackenzie (mountain man) was the self-proclaimed doctor. Using herbs, plants, and other materials, Mackenzie proved to be a healing wonder sought by the sick and injured. A young Indian was brought to his attention who's thumb was severed by a gun, only a piece of skin kept the thumb attached. Mackenzie dressed the wound with the juice from the spruce fir bark and made a poultice from the roots of the spruce fir.

A salve was made from Canadian balsam (oily or gummy oleoresin used for medications), wax, and tallow dropped from a burning candle into water. The salve was used with the dressing. The dressing on the thumb was changed 03-times a day for 01-month, the wound healed completely. The Indian boy was so thankful he went hunting returning with an elk's tongue (delicacy) for Mackenzie.

Through Alexander Mackenzie's explorations, he was elevated to one of the top traders and wilderness leaders in his day. A river was named after him - Mackenzie River. The Mackenzie River located in the Northwest Territories, Canada, flows from Great Slave Lake to the Arctic Ocean and is only navigable from June to October. The Finlay-Peace-Mackenzie river system is the longest in Canada clocking in at 2,635-miles!

Healing Shaman: It DOES NOT MATTER if shamans were stone fakes or not. If their followers BELIEVED in them, then their healing power - fake or not WORKED or had a better chance of working for the follower who indirectly used their own mind to heal their ailment.

Hearne's (mountain man) witnessed some fascinating "tricks" used by shamans. One fascinating trick was a naked shaman completely swallowed a bayonet till he demonstrated pains that the bayonet was presently in his stomach. The shaman then produced the knife pulling it out of his mouth. His naked body could hide no bayonet.

The shaman was demonstrating his healing power particularly to a very sickly man who was bed-ridden. After the shaman consulted with the very sickly man, days later he was able to walk. Days later he ventured to the southwest walking 07 to 08 miles a day. Hearnes also witnessed shamans placing both hands and arms up to their elbows in boiling water without any injury!

Even today, right now, I see evangelist "healing" the sick. Whether on TV or live, they use "shotgun healing" stating something like "...*someone has a severe pain in their right leg...*" No Sh!+! With millions and millions of viewers, odds are somebody has got to have a pain in their right leg!

Then they say *"I command thru the power of God that pain be gone - be gone!"* That one lone viewer in Anywhere, USA BELIEVES the evangelist and God are talking and healing him/her! And guess what happens!

The pain goes away! Is this a real miracle of Mind-Over-Matter! In my humble opinion, God had nothing to do with it. God in his wise ways gave us a body & mind that has the capabilities to heal itself and others!

Like I stated many times before, if you don't BELIEVE, ain't nuthin gonna happen!

Healing Silver: On 22 December 2007, National TV reported a man in California who swears by the healing results of colloidal silver. Since 1993, he's been drinking colloidal silver to cure his malady(s) and he's been drinking it ever since.

One distinctive feature about this man, his face has turned blue. Not from drinking colloidal silver but by rubbing it on his face. Colloidal silver can be purchased at most health food stores or you can purchase your own little machine to make your colloidal silver.

Healing Snake Oil: When you hear the 02 words "snake oil" one thinks fake, scam, worthless, gimmick,... The following comes from different sources concerning the healing power of snake oil. Let me try to give you another take on snake oil - healing snake oil.

a) Dr. Richard Payne: Dr. Richard Payne of Brandine University, _____, extracts potent oils from different species of snakes. Dr. Payne states these snake oils have healing properties and may aid to remedy problems with arthritis, nail fungus, rheumatism, sore muscles, and many more.

b) Phillip Gardner: After "intensive research", Phillip Gardner discovered that the correct SECRET combination of snake venom and blood actually gives the human immune system a super boost that may be unmatched by any herb or drug in existence today.

c) Udo Erasmus: According to the Udo Erasmus author of the book *Fats That Heal - Fats That Kill*, snake oil originally came from China. In the 1860s, Chinese labor railroad workers brought their snake oil from China. Their snake oil comes from the Chines Water Snake – *Enhydris chinensis*.

The Chinese would treat their arthritis, muscle pain,... by rubbing the snake oil into the painful site. It turns out their snake oil is loaded with eicosapentaenoic, also known as EPA which is the king of healing Omega-3 fatty acids. This snake oil can be rubbed-on or ingested. See *The Country Doctor's Big Bag Of Common Sense Cures* in the POC Section.

****

In October 1947, Colonel Dean was ordered to South Korea as a military governor and deputy to Lt. General John R. Hodge who was at that time commander of all American occupied forces. On 15 August 1948, Colonel Dean became commander of the 7th Infantry Division headquartered in Seoul, Korea.

Note: At this time, I believe Colonel Dean was promoted to Major General (01 star). As far as I know, all Division Commanders are Generals.

At this time the 7th Infantry Division was relocating to northern Japan. In May 1949, Major General William F. Dean became Chief of Staff for the 8th Army under commander General Walton Walker.

In October 1949, General Dean became commander of the 24th Infantry Division. On 25 June 1950 the North Korean Army, crossed the 38th parallel invading South Korea and the Korean War began.

General Dean and his unit were scattered and eventually overrun by advancing North Koreans. The fighting got so bad, brave American soldiers who worked in the mess hall, clerks, messengers,... put down their work tools and picked-up weapons. Now they were fighting as infantrymen! General Dean along with other soldiers evaded as best they could with enemy all around them. With multiple breaks-in-contacts, General Dean became a lone evader and was eventually captured. In all of American history, it's very rare to have an American General to be put in POW status. Here is one of many of General Dean's survival tricks as an evader and as a POW.

Healing Sunbath: On 29 October 1951, General Dean was moved again. At his new location he was allowed to take a 45-minute sunbath. Sunning is great as long as you don't overdo it. The sun gives the body Vitamin D.

Here's a quote from the Gettysburg Program: *Vitamin D is needed for calcium and phosphorous absorption and utilization. Necessary for growth, Vitamin D is especially important for normal growth and development of bones and teeth in children. Vitamin D is important in the* **prevention and treatment of osteoporosis, rickets, hypocalcemia as well as enhancing immunity!**

The sun's ultraviolet rays can be converted to Vitamin D by exposing the face and arms to the sun three times a week. Don't overdo exposure to the sun. My research also indicates that obtaining Vitamin D from exposure to the sun **helps with problems of depression.**

Sources of Vitamin D are alfalfa, butter, cod liver oil, dairy products fortified with Vitamin D, eggs, fish liver oils, fatty salt-water fish, halibut, liver, milk, oatmeal, salmon, sardines, sweet potatoes, tuna and vegetable oils.

The sun also helps kill bacteria on the skin's surface. Bacteria that may cause disease.

****

Dr. John Heinerman, author of *Natural Remedies From Around The World*, is a renowned medical researcher. He's authored more than a dozen books and many have been translated into 12 different languages. And his latest book - *Natural Remedies From Around The World* - is worthy of your purchase.

Healing Tea Tree Oil: I like putting items in any survival kit I make (made hundreds) that must not only satisfy the *8 Elements of Survival* (Fire, Water, Shelter, First-Aid, Signal, Food, Weapons, and Navigation), but each item should have multiple uses. And here's an item I may add to my 50-calibre ammo can survival kit - it's a small bottle of Tea Tree Oil.

Why Tea Tree Oil? Tea Tree Oil comes from the leaves of the Australian tree *(Melaleuca alterifolia)*. Tea Tree Oil has been used for hundreds of years and just recently has scientific research backed its effectiveness as both an antiseptic and antibacterial compound.

Tea Tree Oil was proven in laboratory tests to **DESTROY 57 different infection-causing organisms**. And the best part is in most cases only a drop or so is needed to enhance or remedy:

- Accelerates Healing
- Acne
- Anti-Inflammatory
- Athlete's Foot
- Bladder Infection
- Cuts
- Dandruff
- Infections
- Nail Fungus
- Pain Reducer
- Plantar Warts
- Reduced Scarring
- Scrapes
- Swelling
- Toe Nail Fungus

For example, Tea Tree Oil can fight ugly toe nail fungus. Approximately 30 million Americans are afflicted with ugly toe nail fungus. Researchers state that only a single drop each day of Tea Tree Oil on a toe nail affected with nail fungus will eventually have the toe nail go back to its normal state - a healthy looking toe nail.

A 02-fluid ounce bottle of pure Tea Tree Oil made by Herbal Harvest can be purchased at you local WalMart or drugstores for about $5.

WARNING: NEVER NEVER take Tea Tree Oil internally. It's highly toxic and may cause brain damage, kidney damage, liver damage, respiratory failure, coma and death.

For another healing oil that's MORE POWERFUL AND SAFER than *Tea Tree Oil*, you must see *Super Healing Oil Of Oregano*.

Healing Yukky Castor Oil:

Can you give me some general information about Castor Oil?
Castor Oil is extracted from the castor bean plant and it's been used for thousands of years for just about every malady - sickness you can think of!

Castor Oil packs (more on this later) have been used with amazing results that most medical doctors would say is impossible. It is even taken internally. Ask your own physician about the healing qualities and successes of Castor Oil.

He\she may probably just laugh or discredit you and tell you to stay away from that nonsense! You have the right to investigate any alternative - at least look into it.

Many varieties of sickly and deadly maladies have responded positively to the amazing healing qualities of Castor Oil. Castor Oil is a **POTENT CLEANSER - DETOXIFIER!** This means it gives your cleansed body the inherent ability to heal itself!

What is Castor Oil composed of?

Castor Oil is mainly composed of ricinoleic acid. Ricinoleic acid is an unsaturated hydroxy fatty acid. A high viscosity oil, some have described it as a nutritious oil.

It's noted to be an excellent emollient and lubricant as well as demonstrating antimicrobial activities. Below is a composition of Castor Oil:

- Ricinoleic acid-------89.5%
- Oleic acid-----------03.0%
- Palmitic acid--------01.0%
- Stearic acid---------01.0%
- Dihydroxystearicacid--00.7%
- Eicosanoic acid-------00.3%
- Linoleic acid--------00.3%
- Linolenic acid-------00.3%

What is the healing secret to Castor Oil?

Heck, scientist and researchers are still conducting research on water - plain ol' water! I forget the name of the field of studying water - but that's all these scientists and researchers do - study water! And they'll be doing it as long as there is money to finance the research!

To come up with bona fide reasons why Castor Oil works along with hundreds of other alternative supplements and treatments & therapies - well don't hold your breath.

My best advice is to try to go back to the basics which is to use common sense and do what your doctor advises (as long as it works) and ALWAYS keep an open mind to other <u>Alternatives Therapies that are safe and help your body to heal itself</u>!

What are some healing benefits of Castor Oil?

The following is a <u>partial list</u> of reported healing results using Castor Oil packs. For many of the maladies listed below, a Castor Oil Pack on the abdomen has demonstrated remarkable results.

- abdominal problems
- aching feet
- acne
- appendicitis
- arthritis
- back pain
- cancer
- colitis
- constipation
- corns
- ear problems
- edema of the ankles
- esophagus
- flactuance
- gall bladder conditions
- hearing loss
- hernias
- Hodgkin's Disease
- Hyperactivity
- Inflammations
- liver conditions
- insomnia

Can I take Castor Oil internally?

Yes you can. I advise you to read any available materials on Castor Oil (see POC Section) and I HIGHLY ADVISE you to seek advice from your physician.

What kind of Castor Oil should I get and where can I buy it?
Like Olive Oil, INSURE the Castor Oil you do buy is:
a) Cold Pressed
b) Cold Processed
c) NO additives

Follow the recommended dosage and instructions from the label and as per your doctor's instructions.

Heinerman Hodgkin's Disease Cure: The following comes from a man named M. Fox who claims to be a descendent of early 19th century privateers who took their numerous bounties from ship wrecks on Bermuda reefs.

Fox states that seaweed and seafoods like shrimp could reverse (cure) Hodgkins Disease. He stated that iodine rich foods have had success with Hodgkins Disease.

To prove this, a woman in her 50s was diagnosed with Hodgkins Disease and had a short time to live. Her husband called Heinerman and he gave her the remedy above.

The woman's husband gave his wife a core diet of cooked seaweed, boiled shrimp, 08 capsules of kelp every day and a few other seafoods.

Within 60 days, the grateful woman had no trace of Hodgkins Disease!!! The husband and especially the wife were extremely grateful. And I hope you are too.

Heinerman Lyme Disease Tea: Each year (as of 1999) more than 10,000 people are afflicted with Lyme disease. It is found in all 50 states and 18 foreign countries. About 10% of Lyme disease cases become chronic.

Lyme disease is an infection caused by a bacterial spirochete spread by a bite from an infected tick. Lyme Disease may affect several organ systems months or years after the bite. Untreated, the infection may affect the brain, heart and joints.

Lyme Disease is more common in the Northeastern states and to a lesser extent in the Midwest. Signs and symptoms of Lyme disease include chill, fever, fatigue, headache, muscle & joint pain, swollen lymph nodes and a skin rash called erythema migrans.

Erythema migrans is a red circular patch that appears at the site of the bite, usually 03 to 30 days after the bite of the infected tick. Lyme Disease got its name from Old Lyme, Connecticut where the disease was identified.

1st Note: At this time there is a **vaccine** that is 80% effective against Lyme disease called *LymeRix*! The vaccine regimen includes three shots over a 01-year period with possible booster shots in the future! See your doctor about *LymeRix* today. You must still check for those critters during and after your outdoor ventures!

2nd Note: I came across a radio interview from a vaccine expert. He (name unknown at this time) stated tens of thousands of people that received the Lyme vaccine are now worse-off. He stated to stay away from this and many other vaccines. RFIR

Anyway, an African tea may just do the trick to remedy sickly Lyme disease. Take the wormwood herb and boil it into a tea. Add a pinch of salt and lime juice and you got a concoction that may fight the Lyme disease symptoms and may be the disease itself.

3rd Note: Wormwood herbs can be purchased at most healthfood stores. I'm not sure if the herb wormwood is the same species (180+) or in the same family as that of the wormwood herb found in Africa.

High Altitude Weight-Loss Diet: Here's another true weight-loss story. How would you like to lose weight and lose it quickly? And get this - you can eat 03 fat-rich restaurant type meals a day and you don't have to do any exercises - none!!! Sounds crazy uh?

Well I actually lived what I call the *"High Altitude Weight-Loss Diet."* Back 1987 while serving with the US Army Special Forces, our A-Team (Green Berets) deployed to Ecuador. We were at a location that was so high up (near Cotopaxi) that we were unable to do any physical training - we couldn't breathe normally to do any running, any exercise at all.

Every day I ate restaurant meals, had a brewski now & then when off duty and still lost weight very fast. I distinctly remember laying in bed in that hotel room and I was laboring trying to breathe. My body was working extra hard every second - 24-hours a day trying to get the vital oxygen it needed.

Again, we were so high up our bodies weren't use to the lack of oxygen so our bodies were trying extra extra hard to breathe every second 24-hours a day.

I remember having some time off and asked one of the Ecuadorian soldiers we were training to help me shop for some new clothes that would fit me. I wasn't familiar with the small towns nearby. As it turned out, I was not only skinny, I turned even skinny skinny!!! I lived in that environment for about a month or so and lost may be a pound of weight a day and remember I ate fat-laden and sugar-laden foods and did absolutely no exercise – no exercise!!

What I call the *High Altitude Weight-Loss Diet* really and truly works! I would ASK YOUR DOCTOR BEFORE YOU CONSIDER THIS DIET. And NO, Denver, Colorado (Mile High city) isn't high enough (5,680-feet). We were located near Cotopaxi (7,884 feet to 19,344-feet) at an approximate elevation of 9,226-feet.

That's real high and nearly dangerous cause altitude sickness and dangerous epoxy starts at 10,000 feet – if my memory serves me correctly. See Multiple Healing Wonders Of Rebound Exercise.

MOST IMPORTANT NOTE: In my humble opinion (I ain't no bariatric physician) I sincerely believe the "High Altitude Weight-Loss Diet" could GREATLY REDUCE OR BANISH the USA and the world's OBESITY PEOBLEM once and for all.

Think of what this diet could do if you ate super healthy food instead of fat-rich food like I did. I have my own documented PROOF of this unique diet and I CHALLENGE ANYONE TO PROVE ME WRONG!!!! Yes, that includes YOU!

WAIT! Here's why I think the *"High Altitude Weight-Loss Diet"* works. I already told you my body was working overtime to try to breathe even just laying in bed. You ever see folks who stop smoking and they immediately start gaining weight? Well their body is already trying to heal itself from all the years of smoking.

Let me interrupt real quick and let me give you my researched data from the - *"The Gettysburg Program - What You Don't Know May Be Killing You. Your Complete Guide To Better Health And Vibrant Living!"* (full version) - at www.amazon.com. Here's my own *"Intensive Research"* for how your body starts healing itself once you STOP SMOKING:

Smoker's Body Starts Healing Itself: OK, if I quit smoking today, will my health improve? It sure will! It will also save you a great deal of money too, depending on the severity of your smoking habit. The following are some compiled facts of what happens when you quit smoking, from the American Cancer Society and the Center for Disease Control:

- Within 20 Minutes -- Your blood pressure and pulse rate drop to their normal levels and the temperature in your hands and feet will increase to your normal levels.

- Within 08 Hours - The carbon monoxide in your bloodstream will have decreased to its normal level and the oxygen in your bloodstream will have increased to its normal levels.

- Within 24 Hours -- Your chances of a heart attack decrease!

- Within 48 Hours -- Your nerve endings will start re-growing and your smell and taste will be enhanced.

- Within 02 Weeks To 03 Months -- Your circulation will improve, walking will improve, walking will become easier and lung function will increase by up to 30%!

- Within 01 To 09 Months -- Your coughing, sinus, congestion, fatigue and shortness of breath will decrease; cilia will regrow in your lungs, increasing their ability to handle mucous, clean the lungs and reduce the possibility of infection; your body's overall energy will increase.

- Within 01 Year -- Your increased risk of heart disease due to smoking will be cut in half!

- Within 05 Years -- Your risk for lung cancer from smoking will have been cut in half, your risk of stroke will be on the way to being reduced to that of a nonsmoker; your risk of cancer of the mouth, throat and esophagus will be half what it was when you smoked!

- Within 10 Years -- Your lung cancer risk will be that of a nonsmoker and precancerous cells will have been replaced with normal cells.
- Within 15 Years -- Your risk of coronary heart disease will be that of a nonsmoker!

Follow the recommended instructions only as per your doctor's approval.

OK, here's my point, the *High Altitude Weight-Loss Diet* really and the body of a smoker have something in common - both bodies are struggling to survive (entire body) which burns calories, burns fat - 60-seconds every minute, 24-hours a day, 07-days a week, 30-days a month, 365-days a year.

High Mallow Plant: The high mallow plant earned the reputation of a **cure-all plant** because of the high mucilage content in its roots. Naturalists, herbalists, and folk healers prescribed high mallow to remedy all sorts of maladies to include coughing, digestive tract inflammation, nausea, urinary tract inflammation, upper respiratory infection,...

North American Indians made poultices from the plant to remedy insect stings, pains from sores, and swellings.

a) Location: Europe, Quebec - Canada, and from the Dakotas to southwestern United States. Found at abandoned lots, roadsides, and waste lands.

b) Description: A hairy biennial plant that grows up to 03-foot tall. Ascending hairy stems provide long-stalks, downy heart-shaped or kidney-shaped leaves that are deep lobed.

Purplish-pink flowers with veined petals appear from
May to August. Its fruit looks like flattened discs.
It's complimented with large amounts of mucilage.

c) Edible Parts: None:

d) Medicinal Uses: The mucilage may aid in respiratory
infections, and aid in inflammations of sores and
insect stings.

e) Killer Parts: None.

Inuit Cancer Cure: The Inuit reign or reigned in the
Arctic regions of Alaska, Canada and Greenland. Inuit
are World Class cold weather survivors orientated
toward Arctic regions. And part of their big bag of
cold weather survival tricks are fantastic first-aid
and serious illness remedies. And here's how they
remedy killer cancer. Let me give you a little story
to back it up.

Ripley's Believe It Or Not did a 04-minute segment on
this 'believe it or not' cancer cure. OK, here it is.

As a young boy Aajonus Vonderplanitz was a very sickly
boy. He'd have colds and flus that would last 03 to 05
months!! Years later in the late 1960s, Aajonus was
diagnosed with a killer cancer - lymphoma cancer.
Lymphoma cancer is a cancer in the lymphatic system.
The lymphatic system filters out bacteria. Lymph
vessels are located in the underarms, necks,... and may
enlarge to lymph nodes when you're sick.

Aajonus immediately underwent radiation treatments.
The radiation treatments did nothing to stop the killer
cancer. Instead the cancer was spreading. Aajonus
stopped his cancer treatments and travelled the world.

Luckily, he encountered the World Class Survivors of killer cold environments - the Inuits of upper North America (Alaska).

An Inuit tribe learned Aajonus was dying from cancer and they had the cure. The Inuit cure was a diet of raw rotten meat. And Aajonus ate the raw rotten meat that very night. Unbelievably, he woke up the very next morning and already felt better just from one meal of eating raw rotten meat!!!

Aaajonus continued his diet of raw rotten meat and was soon cured of his killer lymphoma cancer that conventional medicine couldn't fix. And to this day (30+ years), Aajonus still eats raw rotten meat to insure he stays super healthy. Aajonus believes in this healing diet. And he's actually a Certified Nutritionist and counsel patients/clients to improve their health.

Jail House Workout: It's called a *Jail House Workout* because of the very confined space in which prisoners exercise in their small cells. You don't need to go to the gym, need fancy exercise machines or have a huge space to workout.

You can do a *Jail House Workout* and do simple exercises like:
- Beat Your Boots
- Flutter Kicks
- Jumping Jacks
- Lifting Weights
- Pushups

- Situps
- Stair Climber (buy a few cheap cement blocks)
- U.S. Army Rifle Drill **(in this book)**

Do these exercises in small sets and workup. Next time you go shopping, take extra extra laps up & down them grocery aisles and walk for 30-minutes pushing your cart. Or go to your local mall and start walking. And don't forget to go up them moving escalators.

Note: Here's my idea I just thought of. Go to the cat section of your local WalMart and load-up on 06-boxes of those 28-pound boxes of Scoop-Away Cat Litter. That's 168-pounds in your cart. Get one of them WalMart Associates to load-up your cart.

Now set your watch and start cruising the aisles doing your own shopping for about an hour. When you get to the check-out, just tell the WalMart Associate you'll buy everything but the cat litter, they'll restock it – it's their job.

Just tell them you figured you didn't have enough money for the cat litter. I figure you just burned at least a few hundred calories & more important burned-up some of that glucose too pushing that cart of cat litter up & down the aisles. See *U.S. Army Rifle Drill Exercises (07)*.
Follow the recommended workout instructions as per your doctor's instructions.

Japanese Diabetes Cure: Guava (*Psidium guajava*) has been used for diabetes for centuries in East Asia. In Japan, Guava Leaf Tea is used after meals to control blood sugar levels.

In a study, people who drank guava tea after eating white rice, their glucose levels were lower than the other group that ate white rice followed by drinking hot water. Guava Leaf Tea can be made using the leaves or you can buy the Guava Tea itself.

Kale The Unknown Super Vegetable: Kale is super vegetable as a potential preventative of several cancers including lung cancer. Noted to be one of the richest of all green vegetables in cartenoids (anticancer agents). A highly nutritious food, spinach has 36 milligrams of cartenoids per 100 grams. However, an equal amount of kale has more than twice the amount of cartenoids (78 milligrams).

Too bad kale isn't a popular food item in the United States and Western countries. A study in Singapore noted that kale, along with common dark-green leafy vegetables like Chinese mustard greens, has significantly diminished the risk of lung cancer!

Kale also demonstrates its ability to prevent atherosclerosis (hardening of the arteries) via a carotenoid called lutein.

In an 18-month study at the University of Southern California, a group of 480 men and women with no history of heart disease were tested for serum lutein.

Those people with the lowest levels of serum lutein concentrations, had a *'five-fold greater increase in carotid artery thickness.'*

According to Dr.Fuhrman (Los Angeles Atheroclerosis Study), kale contains a special protective protein called Nrf2. This Nrf2 and here's a quote:

"It creates a sort of Teflon coating in your arteries to keep plaque from adhering."

Kale may also aid those afflicted with diabetes. Kale has more nutrition values than spinach. Kale could help improve blood glucose control because kale is loaded with fiber.

Studies have shown that a high consumption of fiber lowers blood glucose levels for Type 1 Diabetics and improve blood sugar, lipids and insulin levels for Type 2 Diabetics.

Kelp The Unknown Cancer Fighter: It is noted that Japanese eat great quantities of seaweed. Epidemiologists have noted that Japanese women have a fraction of breast cancer in comparison to American women. Japanese women who are diagnosed with breast cancer live longer than American and British women.

A 1974 Japanese study noted that kelp not only helps prevent the development of breast cancer, but that it could also treat existing tumors! Kelp was instrumental in slowing the progression of breast malignancies in 95% of test animals. Sixty percent of these test animals went into complete remission!

Dr. Jane Teas of the Harvard School of Public Health speculates that the chemical called fucoidan in seaweed may be instrumental in the anti-cancer capacity of kelp. Dr. Teas also notes that seaweeds have potent antibiotic properties.

Researchers at the University of Hawaii School of Medicine in Honolulu noted that a dried version of seaweed, called wakame, helped cure and prevent lung cancer in laboratory animals! These researchers found that the active ingredients in seaweed boosts the immune system! Kelp tablets may available in many health food stores.

Laydon's Burn Remedies: I heard a story of a lady that burned her fingers from hot grease. The burn site (tips of 03 fingers - 1st and 2nd degree burns) was 1/3rd the size of my burn (keep reading). After everything was said and done, the uninsured casualty paid more than **$800.00 of medical bills**.

The morning of 010900C October 2006, I was pouring boiling water in my *Thermos* thermos bottle to make tea. This way I can make twice the amount of tea using only 03 tea bags instead of the recommended 06 tea bags.

By steeping the tea bags in the thermos for a couple hours, I get the same amount of tea for 1/2 the price.

Anyway, I was pouring boiling hot water straight off the stove into my thermos through a funnel. The funnel moved and the hot boiling water poured onto my left hand. It took a second or 02 for the burn to register.

I stopped pouring the hot water on my hand and wrist but I stubbornly still held my thermos so not to spill the contents into the sink. It turns out half my hand and part of my wrist had very bad burns (all red in color) and then the NON-STOP STINGING THROBBING PAIN followed. I initially put some Super PAV ointment on it but the pain didn't lessen a lick. So I went to my A-Z Index to find some home remedies for the burns (all red - [completely burned-off all the skin], swelling and blistering). The following is my own R&D for burn remedies and I even gave them a rating for pain and timeliness.

a) **Super PAV:** Super PAV from NATR IS great topical healer but it does nothing immediately for pain. After a few hours, I took off the Super PAV and then tried *Sensodine Fresh Mint Toothpaste (SFMT)*.

b) **Sensodine Fresh Mint Toothpaste (SFMT):** I have to tell you, this toothpaste works. The pain is 95% gone! I applied a good dose of this toothpaste and gently covered all the areas. Within minutes I started feeling relief and within 30-minutes, the pain is 95% gone. Reapply as needed. What about other toothpastes?

Note: Toothpaste must be a paste not a gel. *SFMT* is green in color.

c) Colgate Cavity Protection (CCP): Colgate has more than a few toothpaste products. You need the **original white paste** toothpaste. Anyway, I removed the *SFMT* by gently rubbing the area under cold water. The *SFMT* had some lasting pain relief even after it was completely removed for it took 06-minutes for the burning pounding pain to return with a vengeance. Anyway, I generously applied *CCP* to the burn site.

In only 04-minutes, I already started feeling pain relief. And like the *SFMT*, 95% of the pain is gone. Reapply as needed.

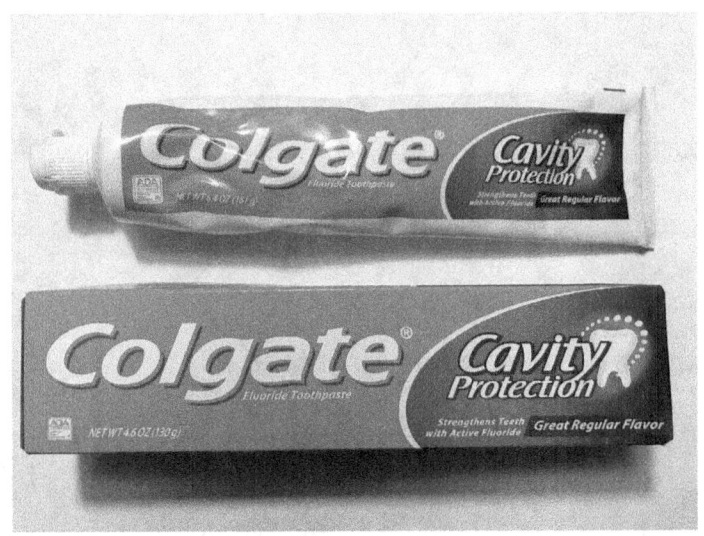

Most Important Note: Under cold running water, I gently removed the *CCP* so to carry-on with the remaining burn pain remedies. After waiting 01-hour, the PAIN DID NOT RETURN! The hand remained somewhat swollen with a little blistering and discolored but the PAIN DID NOT RETURN!

Thus, I discontinued my R&D for I will not deliberately burn myself with boiling hot water. Just to make sure, I reapplied the CCP to insure the burning pain did not return.

However, if you truly want this R&D, send me $50,000.00 and I'll do it just for you!!!! Yes, I'll put everything on camera.

d) Nature's Gate Winter Gel Natural Toothpaste(NGWGNT): The reason I added *NGWGNT* is because I annotated *Toothpaste Fire-Starting* in my Survival Program, you'll learn how I used it to start an emergency fire. Now let's see if we can extinguish burning pain with it. I stated earlier that you should use toothpastes that have paste in them and <u>not gels</u>. *NGWGNT* own name states that it's a gel but let's see if it works anyway.

I liberally applied *NGWGNT* to the burn site and did get some relief but I was still in pain. The *NGWGNT* was better than nothing. Again, see *Colgate Cavity Protection*.

e) Tomato: Slice a tomato and place the fresh slice(s) on the burn site. Repeat as necessary. RFIR.

f) Onion: Slice an onion and place the fresh slice(s) on the burn site. Repeat as necessary. Onion is complimented with antibacterial qualities. RFIR.

g) Potato: Slice a potato and place the fresh slice(s) on the burn site. Repeat as necessary. RFIR.

h) Honey: Liberally apply honey to the burn site. Clean and reapply as necessary. RFIR. You must see *Honey* in the A-Z Index.

i) Acupressure: First degree burns are indicated by a redness of skin. This can be brought on by exposure to the sun, heat, chemicals,...

More serious burns are categorized as 2nd (blisters), 3rd (destruction of skin), 4th (muscle & bone damage & destruction), and 5th degree burns (muscle & bone damage & destruction). This acupressure application is orientated towards 1st degree burns only.

The points are located on the inside of each hand where it meets the wrist and centered on the crease located there. Apply firm pressure. Pain should diminish soon. Repeat application as needed. See Sketch below.

Note: RFIR = Requires Further Intensive Research.

Burn Remedy Pain Definitions!

I divided pain remedy into the following ratings based on pain relief itself and the time it took to relieve the pain.

Excellent Plus---Relieves pain within 30-minutes and initially 90%+ of the pain is gone. Soon after there is 100% pain relief and the pain does not return (01+ hour) even after the concoction is completely removed. Highly recommended.

Excellent---Relieves pain within 30-minutes and 90%+ of the pain is gone.

Good---Relieves pain within 60-minutes and 70%+ of the pain is gone.

Fair---Relieves pain within 90-minutes and 50%+ of the pain is gone.

Poor---Fails to relieve any pain for 03+ hours.

RFIR---Requires Further Intensive Research.

Burn Remedy Pain Ratings!

a) Super PAV: Poor

b) SFMT: Excellent

c) CCP: Excellent Plus

d) NGWGNT: Fair

e) Onion: RFIR

f) Tomato: RFIR

g) Potato: RFIR

h) Honey: RFIR

i) Acupressure: RFIR

You can type or paste your text in here. Pretty cool huh?

Laydon's Healing Spice Concoction: Just to prove to you that I BELIEVE in alternative medicine, let me give you one of my many true stories when it comes to healing myself.

I (author) **BANISHED SEVERE MUSCULAR BACK SPASMS WITH CAPSICUM (CAYENNE PEPPER)!!** While conducting research on capsicum - cayenne pepper (mid 1990s), I decided to see what it would do for SEVERE MUSCULAR SPASMS that

I've ALWAYS had on the middle left side of my back since I can remember - since I was a small scrawny kid. The spasms were so severe, they would literally take my breath away!

One time I was literally paralyzed on my back in my truck and wasn't able to move for 45 minutes! Anyway, this is what I did. My back went out one day (November 1995) so I put some capsicum - cayenne pepper (150,000 SHU) in three capsules. I swallowed them and waited. Now the SEVERE MUSCLE SPASMS that I've had since I was a kid would usually last 10 days to two weeks! Within hours, I really felt relief. Sometimes, I would bend or turn a certain way and the spasms felt like they wanted to flare-up but they didn't!

I went to sleep that night and woke-up the next morning, THE MUSCLE SPASMS WERE GONE! MADE ME A BELIEVER! Since then, I've always supplemented cayenne pepper to my meals! I've NEVER had any more problems with SEVERE MUSCLE SPASMS! Why does it work? I really don't care! All I know is that it does! Beats buying all those EXPENSIVE over-the-counter medicines for $15 a shot. I use cayenne pepper for just a few pennies!

Here's my own UPDATED formula to keep them 'back spasms from hell' away.

Ingredients: 1/3 iodized sea salt, 1/3 black pepper, 1/3 tumeric and a capsule or two of cayenne pepper rated at 150,000 Scoville Heat Units [SHU] (or higher).

I place all ingredients in a plastic container, secure it with the top. I mix it up. I sprinkle the concoction on most of my meals. The core ingredient that keeps the back muscle spasms away is the cayenne pepper. The cayenne pepper must be HOT - at least 150,000 SHU. Why it works? Don't know for sure. I think the cayenne pepper opens up the muscles via the blood so the muscles don't spasm. See *Tumeric*.

Lentils: An international 25-year study that included 12,763 people from Japan, United States and 06 European countries found that legumes like lentils were linked to an 82% reduction in the risk of death from heart disease. Why? Cause lentils include:

- Fiber
- Folate
- Magnesium
- Potassium
- Protein

George Matelijan, the author of *"The World's Healthiest Foods,"* calls magnesium - *"nature's own calcium channel blocker,"* a type of drug that fights hypertension. See *Magnesium*. See *Glycemic Food Index*.

According to the journal - Clinical Nutrition - eating 01 serving of lentils each week can cut Type 2 Diabetes by 33%. Why? Lentils are fiber-rich and have slow burning carbohydrates that keep blood-glucose and insulin levels low. Plus, lentils help you feel full a lot longer, thus preventing you from eating more.

1st Note: I try to conduct more R & D on my 'intensive research' so I went out and purchased 07 01-pound bags of Lentils at $01.54 each for a total price of $10.78 excluding taxes. See photo below.

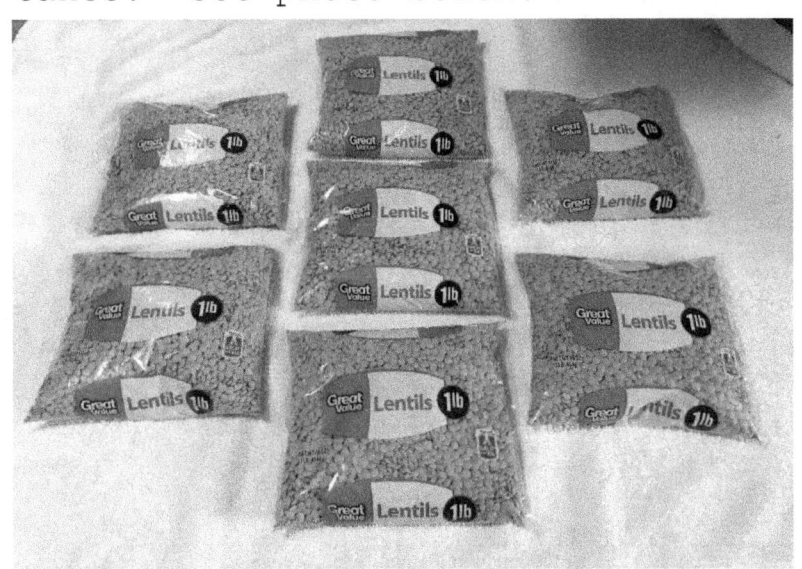

2nd Note: I priced Lentils at www.amazon.com If you want to save money, they offer Lentils in 25-pound and 50-pound bags!!!

3rd Note: I just made a big <u>DELICIOUS</u> meal of lentils and here are the details.

Recipe: 01 medium size pot with lid, 01 spoon, 01 heaping tablespoon of coconut oil (cold), 01-cup of lentils and 02 ½ cups of pure water.

Step 01: Place the lentils in the pot.

Step 02: Pour the water in the pot with the lentils.

Step 03: Add the heaping tablespoon of cold coconut oil.

Step 04: Heat on low heat – simmer – for 30 – 45-minutes. Test the texture to your liking.

Step 05: The lentils will at least double in size. This recipe will provide 02 meals.

Step 06: I added my own concoction to my meal. See *Laydon's Healing Spice Concoction* followed by a couple pinches of sea salt.

Macadamia Nuts: Macadamia nuts offer a bounty of nutritional like calcium, carbohydrates, dietary fiber, monounsaturated fat, polyunsaturated fat, protein, saturated fat, Vitamins B1, B2, B3, B5, B6, B9, C, E, iron, magnesium, manganese, phosphorous, potassium, and zinc.

According to a study from the Louisiana State University, people that ate almonds, cashews, **macadamia**, pistachios and or walnuts, **have a lower risk for Type 2 diabetes and heart disease**.

WARNING: Macadamia nuts are TOXIC to dogs.

Magnet Therapy: Back in the late 1990s I was doing some research on Reflexology. I interviewed a lady at her house in Belleville, IL.

Her husband was there and they both also told me about Magnet Therapy. They showed me these special magnets that have several North & South Poles instead of a regular magnet that has just a single North & single South Pole.

And they had this special material that showed me the many poles of these special metal discs that were the size of a quarter $.25 cent piece.

Her husband told me that he glued some of these special magnets to his gas tank and he got a 25% increase in gas mileage.

He told me the magnets somehow enhance the gasoline so it burns better. I never got around to trying this application to prove or disprove it.

Over the last couple of decades, lots of folks are using Magnet Therapy to improve their health, remedy health problems and more. Golfers wear gloves that have magnets in them to help them in their game. Folks use mattresses that have magnets in the mattress to improve their sleep.

Folks with back problems sit on back & seat cushions to go pain-free. Folks wear wrist, knee, elbow, ankle,… supports to improve their joint health.

'Magnet products' are being used by professional athletes to enhance their performance. That's my warm-up to Magnet Therapy.

Now what about Magnet Therapy when it comes to Diabetes. Diabetics that suffer from diabetic neuropathy in their feet which is long-term damage to nerve fibers from blood sugar levels being too high over several years. Poor circulation results which leads to more problems with the feet. A test of diabetics suffering from poor foot circulation using magnetic insoles, resulted in **90% of the participants had improved blood circulation to their feet**.

Get this, drinking water that has been magnetized by these special magnets (several North & South Poles), may **reverse the effects of high blood sugar levels**. Which affect high cholesterol levels which affects the reduction of plaque on artery walls which affect the reduced chance of heart disease.

Mediterranean Diet: People in the Mediterranean have been noted to develop far less heart disease than Americans, even though they drink, smoke, and even consume as much or more saturated fat than Americans! **What are they doing different?** Their diet consists of an oil they use on their vegetables, grain-rich dishes, and meats. They even dip their bread in it! It's olive oil! Yes olive oil.

One added bonus of monounsaturated fats is they maintain HDL (high density lipoprotein) that helps prevent heart disease. **Olive oil, peanut oil and canola oil are noted to be highest in monounsaturated fats.**

Ensure you read the Nutrition Facts label on any cooking oil. Look for the word *"monounsaturated."* Look for the least amount of saturated fats and the most monounsaturated fats.

WARNING: ENSURE you use *"cold pressed"* olive oil! Use all cooking oils sparingly! Read about *Cholesterol* related data throughout this Survival Book.

Why are people who live by the Mediterranean Diet, healthier than Americans despite their high tobacco consumption, low exercise level, and modest health-care system?

The Mediterranean Diet is a diet low in meat, but high in cereal, fruit, grain, legumes, monounsaturated fats, nuts, and vegetables. Recent French Study found that the Mediterranean Diet after a heart attack was 70 percent more life-saving than the Standard American Diet (low-fat diet-less than 30 percent fat calories). Some Harvard Researchers favor the Mediterranean Diet over the Standard American Diet.

A research effort, called the Seven Countries Study, examined 12,763 men ages 40 through 59 in the Netherlands, Finland, Italy, Greece, Croatia and Serbia, Japan, and the United States.

Ten years after their initial screening, the study reported several important results:

- Mediterranean groups had lower death rates from all causes than the northern European and American groups.

- Lower mortality from coronary heart disease in the Mediterranean countries.

- Men at the peak of their lives (45 years) have longer life expectancies in Greece than in any other European or North American country despite their high tobacco consumption, low exercise level, and modest health-care system.

- The Mediterranean Diet is based on traditional eating patterns evolving over centuries in Greece, Italy, North Africa, Southern France, Spain and several Middle Eastern nations. All share a general pattern of cooking and ingredients. The diet is rich in fruits, vegetables, legumes, and grains. The principal fat is olive oil! Lean red meat is eaten only a few times a month and in small portions.

Eating foods from animal sources - namely dairy products, fish, and poultry is low to moderate. Wine is drunk with meals. Plenty of crusty country-style bread is enjoyed with each meal. The major fat used in the Mediterranean Diet is olive oil! Olive oil is primarily a monounsaturated fat, which is noted to lower harmful low-density lipoprotein (LDL) blood cholesterol and may increase good high-density lipoprotein (HDL) blood cholesterol. Olive oil isn't the only key to a healthy diet. See *French Factor*.

Here are some Mediterranean Eating Tips:

- Switch to olive oil (extra virgin).

- Avoid butter and margarine. There is nothing wrong with putting olive oil on toast or whole grain bread.

- Cut meat consumption. If you do eat meat, ensure it's lean. Try small portions of poultry or fish with plenty of vegetables.

- INCREASE fruit and vegetable consumption.

- Eat plenty of whole grain bread. The darker the better (ingredients not burnt).

- Eat a salad at the beginning and end of each meal.

- Wine at each dinner meal. It's been noted that a couple glasses of wine each day may protect against coronary heart disease. Read about the benefits of red wine in the *French Factor* and see *Special Diets That Heal*.

Mentally Exercising Mind-Over-Matter Trick: Here's a neat Mind-Over-Matter application. As you know I strongly believe in Mind-Over-Matter applications and you can read about em' throughout this Survival Program.

And like I've always said, *"If you don't believe ain't nuthin' gonna happen!"* Here's a Mind-Over-Matter application that's backed-up by a wise researcher and scientific proof!

First of all, your conscious mind knows the difference between what is real life and what is fantasy. But your subconscious doesn't know the difference. That's why many Mind-Over-Matter applications tap into the subconscious so the user does the impossible.

According to Dave Smith, Ph.D,. a sports psychologist at Chester College, England *"We found that the parts of the brain that control movement are stimulated by thinking about movement."* And muscle increases the metabolism which burns calories - fat even when you sleep.

"To a certain extent, the mind (subconscious mind) can't tell the difference between really doing something and imagining it. You need to imagine that you are actually doing something athletic."

Dave Smith, Ph.D., says you don't have to sweat you need to CONCENTRATE. *"Close your eyes and imagine how you'd move your body, what it would feel like."* Dr. Smith states **just 05 concentrated minutes a day should do the trick.** That 05-minutes a day translates into 22-pounds a year! Want proof?

Dr. Smith did a study at Manchester Metropolitan University using 03 groups of people. The 1st group concentrated on muscle contractions 20-times a day for a whole month. The 2nd group actually did the real exercise.

Dr. Smith found that the 2nd group that did the actual exercise, increased their strength by 33%. The 1st group that imagined the muscle contractions increased their strength by 16%! The 3rd group that did nothing increased their strength by 00%.

Now who can use this Mind-Over-Matter application? YOU can! And YOU can do it just about anywhere (except driving or activities that endanger your life or other lives). Try doing it before you go to sleep at night. So try it, **BELIEVE IT**, YOU HAVE TO BELIEVE IT WORKS! Your mind is an AMAZING MACHINE no computer can match! See *Power Of Visualization*.

Mexican Cactus Healer: James H. Cook, a cowboy, guide, hunter, and scout was one of the last to live the life of the Old West before it was gone forever. Shot by a Lipan Indian arrow made from dogwood, possibly poison-tipped, Mexicans came to his aid. To treat the wound, they first pulled the arrow from his calf. They inserted pepper berries in the wound. Then they took cactus leaves, burned off the thorns and secured the hot cactus leaves to the wound.

Note: The cactus used may have been the widely available prickly pear cactus that's loaded with nutrients. See *Indian Gator-Aid (prickly pear)* in the 2004 AASN. As far as the pepper berries, they probably came from a one or more of a variety of chili plants grown throughout Mexico and the world.

Chili contains capsaicin that's already proven as a bacteria fighter, aids in circulation, pain reducer, promotes healing, remedies ailments like bursitis, rheumatism,... That's why you'll see capsaicin in plenty of over-the-counter products.

Mexican Diabetes Cure: According to the team at Children's Hospital in Mexico (August 2002), they reversed diabetes of a 17-year old girl with Type 1 Diabetes.

Up to 01-year after her treatment she needed absolutely no insulin injections or any type of diabetes medicine. What was her treatment? It's called *"xenotransplantation."*

Xenotransplantation is a transplantation from animal to human. What did they transplant? The team of doctors transplanted pig insulin cells from a newborn pig to the 17-year old girl.

Other teenage subjects underwent *"xenotransplantation."* Some responded halfway while others had no response at all.

Multiple Healing Wonders Of Rebound Exercise: What the heck is rebound exercise? I'm going to tell you about an exercise that has proven to be very healthy and very worthy of your attention. It's called rebound exercise.

Rebound exercise is the act of bouncing up and down to exert the right amount of gravitational pull. At the top of the bounce you're weightless. At the bottom of the bounce you're subject to 02 to 04 "Gs" (gravity forces).

So what? Bouncing up & down, what's the big deal? With the bouncing up and down, your 100,000,000,000,000 (01-hundred trillion) cells in your body weigh more due to the Gs.

Because of the Gs, those cells begin a cleansing action at that cellular level and they become stronger. The arteries begin to cleanse themselves too as does the lymphatic system (immune system).

And here's are some more bonuses. Rebound exercise improves the performance of your heart, tones muscles, strengthens skeletal mass, improves energy,...

And since your health improves at the cellular level there's a list of other healthy benefits. Here's a list of some of them:

- Arthritis
- Brain functioning
- Cancer fighter
- Coordination
- Constipation
- Digestion
- Endurance
- Eyesight
- Heart disease fighter
- Immune system
- Lower blood pressure
- Metabolism
- Muscle mass
- Muscle toning
- Osteoporosis
- Premature aging fighter
- Sleep
- Toxin discharge
- Varicose veins
- Weight loss

So you see there are multiple benefits to healthy rebound exercise. And rebounding is a gentle low impact exercise. According to NASA research, our cells live in a zero gravity environment.

But add some G forces to our cells, it aids in toxin elimination and stimulates the Lymphatic system (immune system). NASA found that people that used rebound exercise had **68% better results than people who jogged.**

According to the Institute for Vibrant Health, other rebound exercise machines are inferior. Inferior exercise machines that could cause injuries to the joints (ankles, knees,...) and back injuries.

For a machine that's made just for rebound exercise, see *Institute for Vibrant Health* in the POC Section.

My Super Spice Concoction For Healing & Taste: I've recently (Spring 2018) modified this concoction. I (author) make a concoction of:

- 07 parts black pepper
- 02 ½ parts iodized sea salt
- ½ part cayenne pepper (130,000 SHU)
- 02 ½ parts garlic powder
- 02 ½ parts turmeric powder.

I place it in an airtight plastic container and add about 10 – 15 pinches of this concoction on each of my lunch and dinner meals.

I've used this concoction for decades and I very rarely (01 per every 04 or 05 years) have any more back spasms from hell. See *Capsicum (cayenne)*.

My Family Stopped Eating Sugar For A Year And This Is What Happened: That's the headline dated 11 April 2014. Go ahead and look-up the article. If not, I'll tell you what happened:

- First of all the family found out all sorts of foods were LOAEDED with sugar. Common and tasty foods like baby food, bacon, bread, chicken broth, cold cuts, crackers, mayonnaise, salad dressing, sausages, tortillas,…
- More energetic
- Sugar craving declined
- Sugar-laden products stopped tasting good
- School absentees dropped from 15 a year to 02 a year
- Common illnesses are less frequent
- Recovery time from common illnesses is quicker

Natural Tasty Diabetes Preventor: North American Indians of 150 to thousands of years ago of just about any tribe were for the most part in <u>excellent physical condition</u>.

They ate off the land that provided them meat, insects, fruits, vegetables, fresh pure water and plenty of physical activity. Many Indian tribes are extinct but the ones that have survived are facing serious health issues.

On 141925M July 2004 (Wednesday), 60 Minutes aired a segment on the Unites States southwestern Indians, namely the Pima & Tohono O'Odham Indians who may be, pound for pound, the most obese & sickly Americans in the United States.

Approximately 70% of Indians over the age of 35-years old are obese and afflicted with sickly and killer diabetes.

Why? It's very simple, it's the killer Standard American Diet (SAD) and the snacks and fast foods are loaded with killer saturated fats, salt, sugar,... (see *The Five Deadly Whites*).

The Pima and Tohono O'Odham are dying right before our eyes. Even Indian kids as young as 04-years old are already afflicted with diabetes.

But 01 nun in particular is doing something about it. Sister Martha Mary Carpenter, Principal of St. Peters Indian School has completely banned all sugar from the school. She also establishes a PT (physical training) program for the school kids.

Once they get off the bus when it arrives at school, they RUN! PT is the 1st activity for the kids so they get their metabolisms revved-up before classes.

Another front has been established to fight obesity and diabetes. Indians are going back to eating the way their ancestors ate. Eating various cactus plants, squash, melons and especially the diabetes fighter - tepary beans. See *Tepary Beans*.

Olive Leaf Healer: Here's a quote directly from the Bible (Ezekiel 47:12): *"The fruit thereof shall be for meat, and the leaf thereof for medicine."* The following fact may tell you there is something to the healing wonders of the olive tree (*Olea europaea*).

The olive tree has a <u>long life of 500 years! 500 years!!</u> Under perfect conditions, the <u>olive tree can live as long as 1,500 years!</u>

126

Amazing uh! I don't know if any institute has really studied the olive tree, but somebody should cause in my humble opinion, the olive tree holds secrets that could have humans vibrantly living independently on their own into the 200-year old range.

Now getting back to the olive leaf. The olive leaf (oleuropein) possesses a powerful antioxidant that naturally lowers blood pressure which helps to prevent cardiovascular disease. Oleuropein, a polyphenol is scientifically proven to:

- Anti-inflammatory
- Antioxidant
- Fights Alzheimer's
- Fights arthritis
- Fights atherosclerosis
- Fights cancer
- Fights cognitive decline
- **Fights diabetes**
- Fights high blood pressure
- Fights neurodegenerative diseases
- Fights strokes
- Lower bad cholesterol (LDL)
- Lower blood pressure
- Prevents cancer

See *East Park Research Inc.* for an olive leaf product.

Here's something amazing about olive leaf extract. When oleuropein (olive leaf extract) was given to animals afflicted with tumors, in only 09 to 12 days, the tumors regressed to nothing.

I could add a couple more pages of benefits when it comes to Olive Leaf Healer, but you got the gist of it. See *East Park Research Inc.* for an olive leaf product.

Onions And Its Many Health Benefits: A 1/2 cup of raw onions provide only 27 calories and are inexpensive. Onions are used in just about every dish imaginable, from appetizers to main courses to soups to even jellies.

Onions can be eaten raw, they can be pickled, sauteed, deep fried, boiled, or steamed onions help boost the good cholesterol which is HDL (High Density Lipo-proteins), lower total blood cholesterol, slow down blood clotting, thin the blood, kill bacteria, and may even counteract against some allergic reactions.

Dr. Victor Gurewich, professor of medicine at Tufts University, prescribes and tells his patients to *"Eat onions."* Dr. Gurewich notes that raw, strong onions <u>elevate critical HDL-type blood cholesterol</u>. The typical therapeutic dose is only 1/2 a medium-size raw onion - or equivalent juice - each day.

Dr. Gurewich says that is usually enough to *"dramatically raise"* HDLs (good cholesterol) an average of 30 percent in about 03 out of 04 heart disease patients! <u>In a few cases, HDL levels have doubled or tripled on the onion regimen!</u> He says that raw onions work best because cooking reduces or destroys the onion's power to raise HDLs.

<u>Raw or cooked onion works as a natural anticoagulant to help prevent life-threatening blood clots that may cause heart attacks and strokes!</u>

According to a study in India, test participants were purposely fed fat-intensive meals that raised their cholesterol to dangerous levels, thus increasing the risk of blood clots.

The participants were then given only two ounces of onion, which was added to their diet, and their cholesterol levels were quickly brought within safe limits!

Onions may be a potential source of possible cancer antidotes because of their concentrated sulfur compounds that are able to turn off cell changes preceding cancer growth.

Researchers at the M.D. Anderson Hospital and Tumor Institute have isolated propylsulfide in onions that in tests blocked enzymes needed to activate a potent cancer-causing substance.

Researchers at Harvard School of Dental Medicine discovered that putting onion extract on cultures of oral cancer cells from animals significantly inhibited proliferation of the cancer cells and destroyed some.

As a matter of fact, the National Cancer Institute has funded much research on sulfides in onions and garlic, naming them promising agents in fending off cancer!

Tasty Note: When I cook using sweet onions, I add the sliced onions at the very end of the cooking process. I like the onions still crunchy and not cooked to nothing. Plus, the sliced onions still hold their valuable healthy nutrients.

Papaya Wound Healer: Papaya is also called papaw and they can be found everywhere in the Americas (jungles, stores) and even abroad. Papaya comes from an evergreen tropical American tree that bears a large yellow fruit. Whether it's a slice of papaya fruit or the juice of the papaya, its noted as a first-aid remedy for wounds.

It helps to prevent infection as well as aiding to accelerate healing the wound. First clean the wound with a few slices of papaya and or the juice. Then apply a slice(s) of papaya or the juice itself to the wound site and secure a clean bandage to the site. Reclean and redress as necessary.

If you feel the wound may take weeks to heal and no professional medical aid is available, wet a piece of bread with papaya juice and apply to the wound. The bread will mold and adhere to the wound site keeping the papaya juice in contact with the wound site. Plus, mold has its own healing qualities.

1st Note: Throughout Central & South America, like bananas, lemons,... I've picked papaya fruits fresh off tree and they were MMMmmmmmmmmmmmmm tasty. And again yes, you could find them in just about any grocery store. For you GIs working throughout Central & South America, now you know a great first-aid medicine that heals and you can even eat the tasty nutritious left-overs!

2nd Note: Here's a direct quote from the Gettysburg Program concerning papaya:

** *"Mexican Indians say that papaya has healing powers. A regular size papaya provides only 160 calories, Vitamin C, a significant source of folic acid, fiber and very low in sodium. It is best to pick a papaya when it is just turning yellow. Papayas provide* **healthy digestive properties** *(enzyme called papain) that have a direct tonic effect on the stomach."*

Papaya Foot Healer: The most abused and forgotten parts of the body are the feet. As you read, papaya may be used to treat wounds and papaya can also be used to soften the dry cracking skin of the feet.

Just take a fresh papaya and mash the pulp in your hands and apply a thin layer of papaya pulp to both feet. Let it soak in for about 20-minutes and rinse both feet with cool water and dry. Yes, you can use papaya pulp to other parts of the body.

Patron Saint For Cancer Patients: See *Visualizations Done By Saints.*

Pet Therapy Stress Buster: Many studies have noted that pet owners have less illness, recover from illness faster, and are likely to live longer! Pets actually take care of their owners in more ways than you know. And it's been proven that pets, all kinds of critters, help lower their owner's blood pressure.

1ˢᵗ Note: Stress is bad for your heart. Why? When you're stressed-out, your body releases stress hormones like adrenaline and cortisol. Overtime those hormones get you all excited which affects your entire system in a harmful way. But an immediate action of stress is it gets folks to drink, smoke cigarettes or both to calm you down.

And smoking and drinking are bad for your health. And that drinking leads to domestic fights which brings on more stress, thus more drinking & smoking and even drugs (legal & illegal). See all the other *Stress Busters* in this book.

2ⁿᵈ Note: I know about Pet Therapy. I care for about 80 critters (koi fish, cats and humming birds [seasonal]) every single day.

Pickle Juice Remedy: I read an article in Runner's World (November 2014 - page 54) on how to remedy muscle cramps. According to Kevin C. Miller, Ph.D., an associate professor of athletic training at Central Michigan University, pickle juice may relieve muscle cramps. He gave pickle juice to cramping victims, water to another set of cramping victims, and nothing to other cramping victims. Dr. Miller states *"Pickle juice relieved the cramps <u>in an average of 85 seconds</u>. Something in the pickle juice, besides potassium or sodium, is telling your muscles to relax and stop firing."*

For my own R & D, I purchased a 24 fluid ounce jar of Vlasic Kosher Dill Spears for $02.35 (08 June 2017). The shelf life is about a year (Expiration - 09 June 2018). Every now and then, I suffer from cramps in my calves and feet. So I'll have this jar of pickle juice standing-by in the fridge and will post my own results at a later date. Now let's carry-on with a fascinating healing story using Mind-Over-Matter.

Pickle Juice Update: Today's date is 12 July 2017 (Wednesday). I gotta tell you. I suffer from muscle cramps (calves & feet) and they HURT! I took a small gulp of pickle juice about once a week or so and I didn't have any painful muscle cramps when I'm laying in bed the last 04-weeks. I drank the pickle juice as a preventative instead of waiting for the muscle cramps.

Bottom line, drinking pickle juice to stop or PREVENT muscle cramps **WORKS!** Why? I don't care. All I know is that it works. I still have some pickle juice waiting in the fridge right now and I'll take a swig of it about once or twice a week or more depending how hard I'm working outdoors.

Placebo Affect, The: Dr. Bernard Siegal, author of Love, Medicine & Miracles, revealed in his book the absolute power of the mind via *The Placebo Affect*. Dr. Siegal's patient called "Mr. Wright" was close to death.

Wright was hospitalized and had cancerous tumors in his abdomen, armpits, chest, groin, and neck. His spleen and liver were enlarged and he could only breathe via an oxygen machine. Almost 02-quarts of milky white fluid had to be pumped from his chest.

Wright was simply waiting to die. Waiting to die, Wright learned of a new cancer drug called Krebiozen. Clinical trials would start on terminal cancer patients that had 03 to 06 months to live, but Wright didn't qualify, he had hours may be days to live.

Wright pleaded and begged his doctor for the new drug. Finally, Wight was allowed the new cancer drug. On Friday the drug was administered to the near dead patient.

On Monday morning, his Doctor returned to the ward expecting Mr. Wright to be near death. Instead he was shocked to find his patient was walking around the ward laughing it up - talking with all the nurses.

Wright was immediately examined and they found his tumors has shrunk down to half their size!

Mr. Wright was injected with more of the new miracle drug Krebiozen. Only 02-weeks later, Wright was examined and they found no sign of any of the cancerous tumors in his abdomen, armpits, chest, groin, and neck. Heck, they sent him home - he was cured. Wright was in absolute great health for 02-months.

Two months after he left the hospital, news about the new miracle drug Krebiozen hit the newspapers, radio & TV and the news wasn't good. The effectiveness of Krebiozen was in doubt and this news immediately sent Wright in a relapse and his tumors came back like magic. Wright was back in the hospital.

Wright's doctor explained to him that the old Krebiozen had some problems with it during shipping and not to take it to heart what he heard on the news. He also stated that a new and far more potent Krebiozen (double strength) is on the way.

A day later, Wright was injected with the new and more powerful Krebiozen. Guess what happened?

Wright again made a full recovery - no sign of any cancerous tumors in his abdomen, armpits, chest, groin, and neck! And guess what again? The new and more powerful Krebiozen was only plain ol' distilled water!

But the story doesn't stop there. In a couple days Wright was sent home making a full recovery and was vibrantly healthy for 02-months. Then the AMA (American Medical Association) reported that Krebiozen was *"worthless in the treatment of cancer."*

This news sent Wright to another relapse where he was again hospitalized. Two days later Wright passed away. In my humble opinion, if Wright would have been protected from any negative news about Krebiozen, he'd of lived a long life.

Power Of Touch: Before I go into this application, let me give you some other *"Touch"* applications in the same arena. Let's start with *Therapeutic Touch*.

a) Therapeutic Touch: Therapeutic Touch (TT) is a "laying-on of hands" healing technique created by a professor of nursing for other health care professionals to use to enhance patient care and treatment progress. TT has been noted to date back approximately 15,000 years. With the help of Dora Kuntz a clairvoyant (associate of Otelia Benssten, M.D. - upstate NY), Dolores Krieger Ph.D., created a technique to teach other health care professionals.

Krieger started teaching TT in 1975 in a class at NYU called *Frontiers in Nursing*. Soon nursing students took their new-found skills into hospitals and private practices of medicine, using it on patients who agreed to try *"a little experiment."*

Dolores Krieger's students returned with more and more testimonials to TT's positive effects.

b) Pranic Healing: Pranic healing does not require physical contact. It is a system using off-the-body healing using prana to treat many illnesses. The treatment is not used on the physical body but used on the energy body. Prana is the vital energy found in the sun, air, and ground.

Pranic healing utilizes activated chakras (energy points) that are located in the palms of your hand and other parts of your body. Chakras become sensitive to the patient's energy and an experienced practitioner can scan the patient's energy field to locate blockages, cleanse them, apply new prana, and stabilize the area.

c) Reiki: Reiki is an energy healing system based on ancient Tibetan knowledge rediscovered by a Japanese theologian.

Reiki practitioners transmit energy by a light touch, a gentle placing of the hands in specific positions of the body. Reiki may be used for emotional, mental, physical, or spiritual balancing.

d) Rosen Method: The Rosen Method bodywork combines touch and verbal communication to evoke muscular relaxation. Light to medium touch increases the body's self-awareness. Rosen Method bodywork focuses on muscular tension, the relationship between that tension and the emotions, and the role of breath in creating more space and flexibility in one's physical structure.

The Rosen Method stimulates the parasympathetic nervous system, whose functions include the constriction of the pupils and the slowing of the heartbeat. Circulation is increased.

Warmth and color return to the areas once frozen in fear or pain. Improved circulation relates to increasing range of movement. Mobilized joints allow more synovial fluid to lubricate and nourish surrounding cartilage and connective tissues. The gentle Rosen Movement is ideal for Seniors.

e) SHEN Therapy: SHEN Therapy is a sophisticated system of applying the Biofield (Qi flow) between the practitioner's hands to the regions somatic (body) affect in the patient's body, releasing deeply embedded traumatic emotion in a precise, gentle, non-intrusive and positive way.

f) Shiatsu: A gentle Japanese massage that works on the acupuncture system of meridians, applying finger pressure instead of needles.

g) Reflexology: Reflexology is a specific bodywork technique of stroking or applying pressure to one part of the body in order to effect changes in another part of the body, relax muscles and stimulate the ***body's own natural ability to heal itself.***

There are several techniques under the generic term Reflexology: Hand Reflexology, Foot Reflexology, Zone Reflexology and Body Reflexology.

The Reflexologist uses a map of the body on the soles of the feet and palms of the hand. Massaging these extremities sends an energy signal that stimulates reflexes, automatic nerve impulses connected to specific areas of the body.

Other parts of the body are the ears, head, torso and back also contain reflexes corresponding to the whole of the body.

h) QiGong: Until 1980, this 5,000 year old practice (QiGong), was kept as a secret within families and religious temples. QiGong is an ancient oriental technique which uses movement and breathing to stimulate the natural healing energies within the body. Practiced regularly, it has been shown to enhance overall vitality, reduce the effects of stress and assist in the resistance to disease.

The world's largest medicineless hospital, the Huaxia Zhineng Qigong Clinic & Training Center is located in Qinhuangdao, China. Its founder is Dr. Pang Ming, a Qigong Grandmaster who is trained in both Western and Chinese traditional medicine.

Since its initial practice in 1988, the clinic has treated more than **180 different diseases (100,000 patients+) with a 95% success rate**! Beat that success rate *"conventional medicine!"* The center avoids medicines & special diets and favors exercise, love, and life energy which is known as chi!
How can you look into this alternative practice?

Luke Chan, the first Chi-Lei Master to be certified outside China by the Zhineng Qigong Center, has practiced Qigong and Tai Chi for 28 years. He now practices in the United States! See *Luke Chan* in the POC Section.

QiGong Masters use a form of *"laying of the hands"* to manipulate the energy force - chi for healing.

OK, now that you have a better understanding of "touch" therapies, let me tell you about the outer body, namely the skin so to better understand why "touch" therapies work.

The largest organ of the body is the skin. The average adult clocks-in at wearing approximately 18 square feet of skin weighing about 08-pounds. And on this layer of skin, it's complimented with at least:

Skin: 05-million nerve receptors.

Finger Tip: 1,000 nerve receptors.

Hand: 10,000 nerve receptors.

And throughout the body are a bounty of acupressure points, chakras,...

Whether "touch" therapies address these nerve receptors, chakras, acupressure points,... or a combination of these - touch therapies really works. And for at least 15,000-years one form of touch therapy or another has been used throughout the world.

One of the most famous *"power of touch"* healers was Frenchman Serge Leon Alalouf. Born in Toulouse, France in 1905, Alalouf even as a young boy knew he had the *"power of touch."*

In 1957, Alalouf was accused of practicing medicine. He was acquitted in a court of law. I'm sure the **276,000 written healing testimonials** may have helped acquit him. One of Alalouf's cured patients include King Alfonso XIII of Spain. Alalouf died in 1982 after being hit by a car.

Power Of Visualization: I've been looking into - investigating the *Power Of Visualization* since the 1990s. It turns of Visualization is more popular than ever. OK, let's carry-on with the *Power Of Visualization*.

Visualization is the conscious effort of imagining your desired goal or goals. For example, we'll use golf. Before hitting the golf ball, imagine you're hitting it in great detail.

Then imagine the flight of the ball going exactly where you want it to go. Now imagine the ball hitting the grass and rolling right in the hole. Imagine this scenario a few times before you actually do it.

And believe it or not modern day golfers (amateurs & pros) use Visualization when they play golf. And other sports professionals (football, swimming, tennis,…) use Visualization to enhance their performance.

Now here's a true story of a boy using Visualization.

- **Terminal Brain Cancer**: Some years ago, a boy located on the East Coast was diagnosed with terminal brain cancer. The young boy's doctor told his parents that nothing could be done to save his life. The doctor stated the boy would soon die.

  But the boy's parents didn't accept their boy's fate so they seeked alternative therapies. The parents took their dying boy to the Mayo Clinic located in Rochester, Minnesota. The Mayo Clinic explored and employed alternative therapies.

  A staff at the clinic suggested that the boy might try using his own mind to fight the terminal cancer. A technique called Visualization where the patient sees in their mind - imagines a game-like scenario of good against evil.

  In this case the sickly boy reluctantly visualized a rocket ships zooming around in his head and firing their guns at the *"big, dumb & gray"* cancerous tumor. The sickly boy visualized this scenario, this same scenario frequently for a few months.

Then one day the boy reported to his parents *"I just took a trip through my head in a rocket ship, and I can't find the cancer anymore."* Eventually the boy returned to the hospital and had a CAT scan. It revealed that the young boy was free of any tumor!! There was no trace of any tumor in the boy's head. See *Vision Therapy*.

Here's a partial list of famous people who used the *Power Of Visualization* to attain their minute goals and major goals:

- Arnold Schwarzenegger (Body Builder, Actor, Governor)
- Billie Jean King (Tennis Pro)
- Gabby Douglas (02 time 2012 Olympic Gymnast Gold Medal Winner)
- Jack Nicklaus (Golf Pro)
- Jim Carrie (Comedian)
- Lindsey Vonn (World Class Skier)
- Michael Phelps (23 Olympic Gold Medals)
- Muhammad Ali (World Heavyweight Boxing Champion)
- Oprah Winfrey (Television Host, Actress)
- Peyton Manning (NFL Pro Football)
- Seattle Seahawks Football Team
- Will Smith (Comedian, Actor)

Psoriasis Solar Healer: Psoriasis is a chronic inflammation of the skin resulting in red, scaly patches. According to Dr. Philip professor and chairman at the University of Missouri - Columbia School of Medicine, intense doses of sun could help 95% of psoriasis sufferers. Why?

UV (ultra-violet) rays fight psoriasis. The Dead Sea area in Israel is a magnet for psoriasis sufferers. And the sun also has other benefits.

Multiple Healing Wonders Of Rebound Exercise: What the heck is rebound exercise? I'm going to tell you about an exercise that has proven to be very healthy and very worthy of your attention. It's called *Rebound Exercise*.

Rebound exercise is the act of bouncing up and down to exert the right amount of gravitational pull. At the top of the bounce you're weightless. At the bottom of the bounce you're subject to 02 to 04 "Gs" (gravity forces).

So what? Bouncing up & down, what's the big deal? With the bouncing up and down, your 100,000,000,000,000 (01-hundred trillion) cells in your body weigh more due to the Gs. Because of the Gs, **those cells begin a cleansing action at that cellular** level and they become stronger.

The **arteries begin to cleanse themselves too as does the lymphatic system (immune system)**.

And here's are some more bonuses. Rebound exercise improves the performance of your heart, tones muscles, strengthens skeletal mass, improves energy,...

And since your health improves at the cellular level there's a list of other healthy benefits. Here's a list of some of them:

- Arthritis
- Brain functioning
- Cancer fighter
- Coordination
- Constipation
- Digestion
- Endurance
- Eyesight
- Heart disease fighter
- Immune system
- Lower blood pressure
- Metabolism
- Muscle mass
- Muscle toning
- Osteoporosis
- Premature aging fighter
- Sleep
- Toxin discharge
- Varicose veins
- Weight loss

So you see there are multiple benefits to healthy rebound exercise. And rebounding is a gentle low impact exercise. According to NASA research, our cells live in a zero gravity environment. But add some G forces to our cells, it aids in toxin elimination and stimulates the Lymphatic system (immune system).

NASA found that people that used rebound exercise had 68% better results than people who jogged.

According to the Institute for Vibrant Health, other rebound exercise machines are inferior. Inferior exercise machines that could cause injuries to the joints (ankles, knees,...) and back injuries.

Reiki - I Got The Power: First let me tell what reiki is and let me tell you my true story. Reiki is an energy healing system based on ancient Tibetan knowledge rediscovered by a Japanese theologian. Reiki practitioners transmit energy by a light touch, a gentle placing of the hands in specific positions of the body. Reiki may be used for emotional, mental, physical, or spiritual balancing.

So here's a true story I think you'll like. I'm very confident you got your money's worth in this AASN! But to make sure you get more than your money's worth I want to relate another TRUE healing story to you with respect to my cat named Obsidian (volcanic glass - black male cat).

In the afternoon of 06 July 2011 (Wednesday), I attended a Reiki class and received a Certificate

Of Attunement, meaning I now possessed the healing powers of Reiki.

Reiki means universal life force energy. An energy that is around us all the time. And to grasp – (channelize) that healing energy and transfer to another person or animal to a specific part of the body for healing, that's using Reiki via your hands because there are things called Chakras in both of your hands. To activate this healing energy like me, you must see a Reiki Master.

I wanted the Reiki qualification in case I needed it in an emergency situation Anytime Anywhere when no professional medical care is available.

Anyway, that evening I returned home. Doing the usual house work, I finally rested a bit in the living room. Ol' Obsidian came up to me and jumped on the recliner next to me and started meowing wanting some food. Then I got the idea to try my new Reiki training on Obsidian. You see, Obsidian has always had problems with his skin / fur. He doesn't have a shiny smooth coat of fur like his twin brother Obama. He's always scratching his itching fur.

Well I activated both hand chakras as taught in class. I grabbed Obsidian and placed him in my lap and secured him with my left hand. I then hovered (not touching him) my right hand over Obsidian's back.

Instantly Obsidian kept looking back behind him like I was touching him or pulling on his fur. I kept hovering my right hand over him (not touching him) and he kept looking back to see what was going on.

This was my proof that the power of healing Reiki really works because Obsidian could actually feel the energy flowing from my right hand into his body.

He repeatedly kept turning around because he could feel something happening on his back. **You might fake it with a human but not with a cat!!!** This is my absolute proof that reiki really works!

I highly recommend that you get a book on Reiki and read the whole book. If you think it's for you, look-up a local Reiki Master and make an appointment. I think I paid only $50 for the whole initial process and you're Reiki qualified forever.

MOST IMPORTANT NOTE: When my Mom was sick with cancer. We hired a Reiki Master to apply her 'magic' to help my Mom feel better. The Reiki Master came in the house.

She wanted the dining room table cleared and blankets place on the table. She also had her own music to play while she applied her 'magic.' We lifted my Mom on the dining room table and the Reiki Master wanted all of us the leave the room.

About an hour later, the Reiki Master said she was done and we lifted my Mom off the dining room table and back to the sofa. I remember this next part distinctly.

After the reiki therapy and days later, my Mom was feeling better and seemed to be more active. I regret no inviting that Reiki Master back to the house for more reiki applications. Again, look into Reiki Therapy for yourself. See *Power Of Touch*.

Richard Quinn's Heart Disease Cure: In his book, *"Left for Dead,"* Richard Quinn, relates a fascinating true story. He was struck with a heart attack which was followed by bypass surgery. The bypass surgery was supposed to *"make him as good as new."*

Well it didn't and his cardiologist stated, *"there is nothing more we can do."* After months of moping, Richard Quinn took some advice from a friend. Richard purchased only 69 cents of cayenne pepper (red), filled several capsules and swallowed them!

The very next morning, Richard Quinn got up and shoveled 04-feet of wet snow off his 28-foot porch! That happened in 1980. Richard Quinn studied the medicinal values of herbs and launched his own company *"Heart Foods Company Inc."*

Read Richard Quinn's book, *"Left for Dead"* at your local library, purchase it at your local bookstore, or order it from R.F. Quinn Publishing Company by calling 1-800-283-3998 or 1-612-924-3525.

His book is packed with information on cayenne pepper and other herbs. See *Capsicum (cayenne)*. See *My Cure For Back Spasms From Hell*.

Saliva Healings And Cures!

Here are a few healings and cures using saliva. Let's start with *Devil Dog Licking Cure*.

Devil Dog Licking Cure: I've repeatedly said over the years that saliva (man & critter) has healing qualities and here's more proof from Africa. This true story comes from an article from Smithsonian magazine (April 2007). Africa's Wild Dogs, also known as devil dogs, painted dogs,... These wild dogs once roamed 3/4 of Africa and numbered in the hundreds of thousands. Very social animals they live in groups of 02 to 30. Today, they clock-in at only 5,000 in number.

The "intelligent" African Wild Dog is noted to be better hunters (day & moonlight hunters hunt in packs launching coordinated attacks) than lions or leopards and have a notable high kill rate. They clock-in at 50-70 pounds and are recognized by their big & round Mickey Mouse ears. But don't be fooled about their size or their cute Mickey Mouse ears for these very fast and intelligent dogs can viciously bring down prey (keep reading - see Item 217) as large as the 500-pound kudu bull (antelope).
Not only are they savvy hunters, they can doctor-up each other too. At one time, a wild dog was viciously swatted by a lion. The lion opened a deep gash to the wild dog's neck area. The vet on the scene took a look at the severe wound and advised that the wild dog be put to sleep.

Nothing could be done to save the wild dog. But his family of dogs knew better. They literally dragged the half-dead severely injured dog back to their den. There they licked the wound constantly. The dog was fed and licked constantly.

After 03-months of nursing, the dog was back with his family and at 100%!!! Now tell me saliva doesn't work to heal wounds!

Licking Cure: I want to tell you about some emergency first-aid used on Army Air Corps Staff Sergeant Ray C. Hunt. On 08 December 1941, Japanese forces attacked the Philippine Islands. US and allied forces eventually surrendered.

SSG Ray C. Hunt, a POW, participated and escaped from the famous Bataan Death March. Evading the Japanese, he luckily found a safe haven with Filipino civilians. Half dead they nursed him back to health.

SSG Hunt initially weighed in at more than 160-pounds. Having survived the fighting and now on the Bataan Death March, he weighed in at about a skinny and sickly 100 pounds. Lost, he wandered into a village half dead.

They fed him and let him bathe. SSG Hunt's foot was in bad shape with a throbbing painful ulcer. The ulcer spread drilling a hole in his foot down to the bone.

With decaying flesh around it, it smelled terrible.
The Filipino family had a dog who came over to smell
the wound. The dog attempted to repeatedly lick it but
SSG Hunt kept kicking the dog away with his bad foot.

The Filipino woman saw this and urged him to let the
dog lick his wound and so he did. The dog's licking
hurt like crazy but he tolerated the extra pain. As
days passed with more licking by the dog, SSG Hunt was
surprised that the ulcerous wound started to heal and
heal fast - solely by the dog licking the wound!

In a week he saw remarkable healing progress! Now you
know your dog is more valuable besides being a friend
and chasing those 9-life critters; your dog could also
be a healer!

Why did this work? I told you how animals lick their
own wounds and wounds of family critters cause their
saliva contains an antiseptic (destroys disease-causing
microorganisms). Make sense huh! The dog's saliva
contains an antiseptic.

Does human saliva contain antiseptic? I don't know but
I would bet it does - RFIR.

Guayaki Saliva Cure: How many times have I related the
possible healings using your own saliva? Well, more
than a few times. Anyway, Guayaki Indians (Paraguay,
South America) used saliva as one of their medicines.

But the best healing saliva came from pregnant women. Why pregnant women? Cause they carry more immune system chemicals that fight-off disease and foreign bodies that may bring harm to the body, especially the unborn child. Anyway, the Guayaki pregnant woman will take her saliva and smear it over the infected area. The saliva is noted to be very potent. See *Licking Cure*. While I'm talking about those survival experts in their specific part of the world, let me tell you about *Guayaki Fat Cure*.

Guayaki Fat Cure: The jaguar was greatly respected for it stalked man to include a lone Guayaki Indian (Paraguay, South America) and the results were a feast for the hungry jaguar. However, the expert predator was also stalked and eaten by the Guayaki Indians. Its meat was a delicacy. But its fat was used as a proven medicine. Jaguar fat was saved and used to remedy all kinds of pains relating to bones throughout the body. We know these common pains as arthritis, condomillatia and rheumatoid arthritis.

I told you about animal fat, because animal fat from various animals has been used and is used for emergency first-aid.

Salmon: Salmon is low in saturated fat and high in Omega-3 fatty acids. Salmon provides only 233 calories per 04.5 ounce steak and only 06 grams of fat per 03 ounces.

Delicious salmon offers the following unique healthy ingredients:

- **CoQ10:** Use caution when purchasing CoQ10 because not all products are offered in its purest form. CoQ10's natural color is bright yellow\orange and has very little taste in the powdered form. CoQ10 should be kept away from heat and light since pure CoQ10 will deteriorate in temperatures above 115 degrees Fahrenheit. Sources of CoQ10 are mackerel, salmon, and those tasty sardines. Sardines contain the largest amounts of CoQ10. See *Coenzyme Q10 (COQ10)*.

- **Selenium:** Sources of selenium may be found in Brazil nuts, brewer's yeast, broccoli, brown rice, chicken, dairy products, liver, onions, salmon, seafood, tuna, vegetables, and whole wheat health-food stores.

- **Vitamin D:** My research also indicates that obtaining Vitamin D from exposure to the sun helps with problems of depression. Sources of Vitamin D are alfalfa, butter, cod liver oil, dairy products fortified with Vitamin D, eggs, fish liver oils, fatty salt-water fish, halibut, liver, milk, oatmeal, salmon, sardines, sweet potatoes, tuna, and vegetable oils.

- **Polyunsaturated Fat:** According to Paul Caldron, D.O., a clinical rheumatologist and researcher at the Arthritis Center in Phoenix,

"A vegetarian diet is good, because the goal for arthritis sufferers is to cut as much saturated fat from their diets as possible and replace it with more polyunsaturated fat." Speaking of polyunsaturated fat, one of the best sources is cold-water fish like <u>salmon</u>, sardines, and herring.

- **Omega-3 fatty acids:** Omega-3 Fatty Acids are made up of two components DHA & EPA! DHA which stands for docosahexaenoic acid. EPA stands for eicosapentaenoic acid. These two nutrients found in Omega-3 are noted to <u>protect against heart disease, stroke</u>, depression... See *"You Gotta Have Your Omega-3 Fatty Acids For Lunch And Dinner!"*

Special Diets That Heal: Diet is a <u>KEY FACTOR</u> in both the prevention and treatment of common illnesses, as well as chronic degenerative diseases such as arthritis, cancer, diabetes, and <u>heart disease</u>. Below are a few diets you should know about:

- **Pritikin Diet** -- In the 1970's, Nathan Pritikin made news with his Pritikin Program that could detour high blood pressure and high cholesterol from reaching dangerous and deadly levels. The Pritikin Program included a low-fat, low-calorie, low-salt diet with a moderate daily exercise program.

893 Pritikin Program participants were studied by a team from Loma Linda University. The 26-day Pritikin Longevity Center program demonstrated there was something to this unique program.

1. 83% were able to terminate their prescription of high blood pressure medicine!
2. Overweight participants lost an average of 13 pounds!
3. Cholesterol levels dropped an average of 25%!
4. **50% of diabetics were able to stop taking insulin!**
5. Participants performed better on mental ability test!
6. Many people were alleviated of their tiredness and required less sleep!

- **Gerson Diet** -- In 1919, Dr. Max Gerson developed a diet to eliminate his own migraine headaches. The Gerson Diet consist of foods that are low in fat, grain & protein products while utilizing large amounts of fresh, raw vegetable juices and other raw foods. Dr. Gerson found that through his research, he discovered not only did this diet eliminate his migraine headaches, but most other health problems like arthritis, **diabetes**, and even terminal cancer!

- **High Altitude Weight-Loss Diet:** See *High Altitude Weight-Loss Diet*.

- **Paleo Diet** – Eat like our ancestors. See *Paleo Diet*.

- **Raw Food Diet** -- Probably the BEST DIET I've come across is the Raw Food Diet. This diet consists of raw fruits & vegetables and juicing. This diet is similar to the Gerson Diet, with the exception of consuming large amounts of grain. This diet has literally solved a wide variety of health problems where conventional medicine has FAILED! Yes, even terminal cases! See *Juicing Therapy*.

- **Mediterranean Diet** - See *Mediterranean Diet*. See *Fasting*.

Spinach: A cup of raw spinach furnishes only 12 calories, whereas a cup of cooked spinach furnishes only 42 calories. Spinach is very low in fat, furnishes Vitamin A as carotene, Vitamin C, Vitamin E, calcium, iron, and many other nutrients.

Spinach provides that much needed fiber to help prevent cancer and helps to lower cholesterol, lose weight, and control diabetes!

According to Dr. Richard Shekelle, an epidemiologist at the University of Texas, spinach has it all including the ability to rev up the metabolism.

According to the Journal of American Medicine, spinach is called *'King of Vegetables.'*

One of many dark green vegetables, spinach tops the list (along with carrots) of foods eaten most often by people worldwide with lower rates of all types of cancer, especially cervical, colon, endometrial, esophageal, laryngeal, lung, pharyngeal, prostate, rectal, and stomach.

Spinach provides high amounts of chlorophyll, which is a noted cancer blocker. Italian studies found that spinach, in test tube tests, was dramatic at blocking the formation of one of the most powerful carcinogens known - nitrosamines.

Of the foods tested (carrots, cauliflower, lettuce, and strawberries), spinach juice was by far the most potent!

Spinach contains folic acid, which is noted as a mood booster. Are you suffering from depression? Eat spinach!

An amino acid called homocysteine found in the blood is noted to increase the risk for heart disease. To counter homocysteine levels, Doctor Havala Hobbs at the University of North Carolina at Chapel Hill, recommends a cup a day of dark green leafy vegetables like spinach.

Super Healing Oil Of Oregano: Here's an exceptionally long list of what oregano kills (bad guys), as well as its benefits for ameliorating a wide variety of disorders.

And this isn't a complete listing either. Odds are YOU or someone close to you is troubled by one or more of the following health maladies and should take a closer look at super healing oil of oregano.

Note: DO NOT mix-up oregano oil with *Oil Of Oregano* - different oils as far as healthy healing. Anyway, as I've always said *"Try the least intrusive method(s) first to remedy your health problem before going forward with conventional medicine of drugs and/or surgery."*

OK, here's the list - oh, see your doctor before using Oil of Oregano:

- Acne
- Alcoholic Neuritis
- Allergies
- Animal Bites
- Arthritis
- Asthma
- Athlete's Foot
- Back Pain
- Bad Breath
- Bed Sores
- Bladder Infections
- Boils
- Bromidrosis (body odor)
- Bronchitis
- Bruises
- Burns
- Bursitis
- Candidiasis
- Canker Sores

- Cellulitis
- Chicken Pox
- Cholera
- Colds
- Cold Sores
- Colitis
- Congestion
- Constipation
- Cough
- Crohn's Disease
- Croup
- Dandruff
- Dengue Fever
- Dental Cavities
- Dermatitis
- Diaper Rash
- Diarrhea
- Diphtheria
- Diverticulitis
- Ear Aches
- Ear Infections
- Ebola
- Eczema
- Emphysema
- Encephalitis (includes West Nile virus)
- Esophagitis
- Fatigue
- Fingernail Fungus
- Flactuence
- Flu
- Food Poisoning
- Frostbite

- Frostburn
- Gastritis
- Genital Herpes
- Giardiasis
- Gonorrhea
- Gout
- Gum Disease
- Hantavirus
- Headaches
- Hepatitis
- Hiatal Hernia
- Hives
- Impetigo (skin infection)
- Ingrown Toenail
- Insect Bites
- Irritable Bowel Syndrome
- Jock Itch
- Kidney Infection
- Kills Amebas
- Kills Antibiotic-Resistant Super-Germs
- Kills Bacteria
- Kills Camphylobacter
- Kills Clostridium
- Kills Cryptosporidium
- Kills Cyclospora
- Kills E. ColiKills Enterobacter
- Kills Fleas
- Kills Flukes Cholera
- Kills Fungus
- Kills Germs
- Kills Giardia
- Kills Lice

- Kills Parasites
- Kills Salmonella
- Kills Shigella
- Kills Ticks (my R&D)
- Kills Viruses
- Kills Worms
- Kills Yeast
- Laryngitis
- Leaky Gut Syndrome
- Leg Cramps
- Listeria
- Low Blood Pressure
- Lower Lung Conditions
- Lyme Disease
- Malaria
- Measles
- Mumps
- Nail Fungus
- Neuritis
- Open Wounds
- Oral Lesions
- Paronychia (nail infection)
- Peptic Ulcer
- Pneumatic Conditions
- Pneumonia
- Poison Ivy
- Poison Oak
- Poison Sumac
- Psoriasis
- Prostate Disorders
- Prostatis

- Pruritus (itchy skin)
- Radiation Injuries
- Rash
- Ring Worm
- Rosacea (face rash)
- Scabies
- Seborrhea
- Shingles
- Sinusitis
- Skin Cancer
- Sleeping Sickness
- Sore Throat
- Spider Bites
- Spinal Infection
- Splinters
- Sports Injuries
- Stomach Disorders
- Sunburn
- Tartar
- Tendinitis
- Thrush (mouth infection)
- Tick-borne Illness
- Tooth Abscess
- Toothache
- Tonsillitis
- Tuberculosis
- Upper Respiratory Tract Conditions
- Urinary Infection
- Varicose Veins
- Venomous Bites
- Vitiligo (skin pigment)
- Warts

- Wounds
- AND MORE...

Super Powerful Subconscious Mind: I have this saying:

"At The Conscious Level We Are Idiots
As Compared To The Subconscious Level -
We Could Be Super Human!"
Joseph A. Laydon Jr. - 1998

In my humble opinion, the subconscious mind could be (if tapped into) the Mother of all Mind-Over-Matter applications.

Did you know that your **POWERFUL SUBCONSCIOUS MIND** can process **20,000,000 to 40,000,000 bits of information per second!!!** Whereas your conscious mind can only process a lousy retarded 40 bits of information per second.

All the other Mind-Over-Matter applications in this book are powerful applications in their own right.

But if you can learn to tap into your subconscious anytime you want, I'm sure you will see great results.

In my humble opinion, most people (97%) are programmed to be and remain unsuccessful throughout their life. I'm not saying most people are programmed to be failures but are programmed to remain unsuccessful, meaning they are not achieving spectacular results in their life.

I think on the conscious level, a person can reprogram themselves. But reprogramming at the subconscious level goes to the core of your being which could provide better and longer-lasting or permanent results.

I myself (author) have been looking into the *Super Powerful Subconscious Mind.* But you have to understand I'm on the pessimistic side. I'm not into wishful thinking. I'm not a supporter for *'The Secret.'*

As you already read or will read of my own accounts concerning Mind-Over-Matter, I KNOW FOR A FACT it can be done, it works. But whether you believe Mind-Over-Matter works or not, bottom line, I believe it's **ACTION ACTION ACTION** that counts.

Getting back to the *Super Powerful Subconscious Mind*, but wouldn't it be worth looking into the power of the subconscious if it could help you out for the rest of your life?

Tasty And Healing Avocados: Avocados have gotten a real bad rap. Heck they're nicknamed *"butter pears"*! Let me give you the healthy facts on those very tasty avocados that could help you fight killer heart disease, stroke, and deadly cancer.

A fat-laden avocado provides a whopping 300 calories, 30 grams of fat (HDL), soluble fiber, potassium, and a dose of Vitamin C, and Vitamins B2 and B6. All the B Vitamins aid to maintain healthy eyes, hair, liver, mouth, muscle tone in the gastrointestinal tract, nerves and skin.

B-Complex Vitamins are coenzymes involved in energy production. B-Complex Vitamins may be useful to combat depression or anxiety. The B Vitamins should be taken together.

Most of the fat in avocados is the healthy fat (monounsaturated). It's the same good healthy fat found in olive oil and a variety of nuts. According to a study at the Instituto Mexicano del Seguro Social located in Mexico had 45 volunteers add avocados to their diet. After a week, the avocado-eating volunteers recorded a "significant drop" in total cholesterol and triglycerides. And at the same time their HDL levels increased.

And avocados may help prevent deadly cancer. According to the Director at the UCLA Center for Human Nutrition, avocados are loaded with glutathione which is an antioxidant that fights disease causing free radicals. Avocados have 03-times as much glutathione than any fruit.

Note: Monounsaturated fats (good fat) help lower bad LDL cholesterol, blood pressure and protect the arteries from arteriosclerosis (clogging of arteries). Monounsaturated fats are found in foods like **avocadoes**, canola oil, olives, olive oil, peanuts, and peanut oil.

Tepary Beans: White and red tasty tepary beans are grown on the flood plains. Like all desert vegetation, they have a unique way of resisting the hot desert heat.

Great food to fight diabetes and for diabetic patients because it helps avoid those sudden spikes in blood sugar. See *Indian Gator-Aid* and *Prickly Pear Cactus*.

165

Thais Don't Get Blood Clots: The Thais (Thailand) use capsicum chili peppers as a seasoning and as an appetizer with their meals.   Their blood is infused with chili pepper compounds several times a day.

Thais physicians have for some time credited regular consumption of chili peppers as the reason that thromboembolism (life-threatening blood clots) are rare among Thais compared to Americans!

German researchers as early as 1965 found chili peppers beneficial for the blood as a fibrinolytic (clot-dissolving) stimulant.   After more testing, Sukoon Visudhiphan, M.D. and his colleagues at the Siriraj Hospital in Bangkok suggested that the frequent stimulation of the clot-dissolving mechanism by chili peppers helps keep the Thais immune to thromboembolism (life-threatening blood clots)!

I (author) always add cayenne pepper to all my lunch and dinner meals.   See:
- Capsicum (cayenne)
- My Cure For Back Spasms From Hell
- Richard Quinn's Heart Disease Cure

The Amazing Healing Benefits Of QiGong: QiGong has been used for more than 5,000 years and may be one of the most powerful hidden alternative therapies ever known.

In China, qigong is vital to the countries health care system. It is not only practiced by 200 million Chinese every single day, it is practiced by millions of others all over the world. Doesn't matter if you're young, old or disabled, something is going on and beneficial with this ancient alternative therapy.

QiGong is a combination of gentle movements, breathing and meditation to improve blood circulation (blood rules), enhance the immune system and get the vital flow of energy known as qi to flow freely throughout the body.

Again, if you don't believe in QiGong and the invisible energy known as qi it ain't gonna work! So let me tell you more about QiGong and this invisible energy known as qi.

QiGong involves the practice of simple gentle exercise movements involving special breathing to complex movements where heart rate, brain wave frequency and other major organ functions can be altered by the QiGong practitioner.

QiGong is noted to stimulate as well as nourish the practitioners body with qi - qi that can break down energy blockages which in turn promotes blood flow (blood rules) and fires-up the practitioners immune system.

The practice of QiGong activates the electrical flow throughout the body - your entire body is a very complex circuit board. Block any part of that circuit board anywhere on your body and you got pain, lack of movement, lack of function and or disease.

Now with the energy of qi also called a universal life force - one could heal the body starting at the cellular level.

"Every cell of your body needs nutrients and oxygen. And there are a lot of cells in your body aching for precious fuel... there are 100,000,000,000,000 (01-hundred trillion) cells in your body."

I've already told you that your body has the inherent ability to heal itself. Sometimes it needs a little nudge from one or more of the 60 Alternative Practices. You decide - it's your call -it's your body. If you're interested in practicing the gentle exercises of QiGong, your local library or your video store may have videos on QiGong.

Healing & Self-Defense

Now QiGong is not only known for its healing gentle exercise but it is used for healing and self-defense! QiGong Masters are using QiGong to heal their patients of sickly disease. They're using the universal life force - qi - and transferring it from their own body to parts of the patient's body where the flow of energy is blocked. This type of healing is not only practiced by QiGong Masters it is learned and practiced by ordinary folks like you and I. It's called Pranic Healing.

Pranic Healing is using this universal life force that is present in your body, ground, air, plants... and people are actually using it to heal themselves and their patients. But guess what? If you don't believe it doesn't work ain't nothin' gonna happen!

As a matter of fact, if you believe it works it will work even though 100-years from now they find its worthless! Then why did it work anyway? Cause YOU BELIEVED IT WAS GOING TO WORK AND IT DID. In the POC Section I'm going to give you the #01 source to learn Pranic Healing from the Master himself.

Yes, they do seminars throughout the US and the cost is a few hundred dollars per person. If you want the ability to heal using *"laying of the hands"* you ought to look into Pranic Healing. Now what about using QiGong or this qi for self-defense?

I have several documentaries of Master and novice martial artists harnessing this "qi" to not only strike with great power at their opponent, break huge blocks of ice, multiple pieces of wood, but also use this "qi" to neutralize the vicious unblocked powerful punches, strikes, kicks to the practicing martial artists.

I have undoctored documentaries of 250-300 pound football players striking these martial artists in the groin, throat, chest with everything they got and failed to hurt the martial artists using "qi" to neutralize the strike.

The vicious strikes should have easily rendered the person on the ground, incapacitated and in the hospital for immediate medical attention especially the martial artist who took the vicious strikes directly to the throat. If they faked it, I don't know how.

At this time, this subject needs RFIR. If I find a source that offering a homer-study course to teach self-defense using this "qi", I'll let you know in a future AASN (Newsletter).

So now you know the powerful healing, and self-defense applications of QiGong and Qi. If you're interested, consider getting your own video to practice these gentle exercises in the privacy of your own home. See POC Section.
Follow the recommended dosage and instructions from the label and as per your doctor's instructions.

The Five Deadly Whites:

What are the Five Deadly Whites (FDWs)?
The five deadly whites are (listed in order as the most dangerous threat to your health): Meat, Dairy, Salt, Sugar, and White Flour.

- **Meat** - Meat contains fat and fat is already linked to many cancers, heart disease, stroke, and diabetes... Meat eaters consume over 50 pounds of fat (cholesterol) each year!

- **Dairy** - Pasteurized milk changes the calcium to an inorganic form which can not be assimilated by your body. Animal products are noted to be sources of LDL (bad cholesterol).

- **Salt** - Your body needs sodium but the sodium chloride (table salt) may be toxic to your body!

- **Sugar** - Sugar is linked to a wide variety of health problems and noted to hinder your immune system.

- **White Flour** -- White flour is missing most of the good ingredients prior to its processing. It's bleached, synthetic Vitamins added, and it's called *"enriched."* Remember the saying *"The whiter the bread, the sooner you're dead!"*

The Missing Trace Mineral That Heals: I've already covered international health survival used by international REAL SURVIVORS throughout this Newsletter; now I want to cover one more unknown super healing trace mineral you have to know about - Indium. So you better understand this unknown and very important trace mineral, I'll use Q & As for this segment.

What is Indium?

Indium is a trace mineral meaning it's needed by the body in very very small amounts as compared to sodium and dozens of other minerals. Indium is Element #49 on the Periodic Table of Elements.

It's a soft mineral, which does not dissolve in water unless compounded (other elements added). It's 99.99% pure, and is the 10th most scarce element of all available elements. Indium was discovered in 1883.

So, what's the big deal about Indium?

Indium is a natural trace mineral and in recent years, is proving to be a leading mineral to fight aging, reverse aging, fight and ameliorate diseases of all kinds,...

For centuries, thousands of years, ancient cultures have used minerals to fight ill health and stay healthy. Like the Chinese and other cultures have used mineral-rich seaweed.

Greeks used iron enriched water. Pioneers drank rusty water for their iron. As I stated, lacking consumption of water, minerals (74+), fat, and other nutrients while in a wilderness environment - you're asking for trouble and you're going to get it quicker than you think - especially in a dry super hot environment and in a super frigid cold environment.

Your body's functioning is going to fade, then simply shutting down (DEATH). Indium is called *"the missing trace mineral."* Until recently has its supplementation to the daily diet been linked to helping the body heal itself and according to the manufacturers, all it takes is 01 single drop a day.

What's the healing secret behind Indium?
Indium, a rare trace mineral through its unique
ingredients helps the body improve its own health in
many ways (keep reading). And it somehow gets the body
to absorb MORE of other trace minerals as well as
recycle them through the body again thus helping the
body perform at peak performance. Like I said before,
your body is mostly made-up of water and minerals
(74+).

Indium levels in the soil and human bodies were found
so low, that even special recording equipment was
unable to record any traces of indium. That may
indicate indium may not be needed to sustain life, but
aid in vibrant health. Just 01 single drop of indium
per day, has recorded many many healing testimonials
across the globe.

Can you give me some healing accounts of Indium?
Sure, there are many, but here's an abbreviated
listing:
- Alzheimer's Disease
- Acne
- Allergies
- Anti-Aging
- Anti-Depressant
- Backache
- Blood Sugar Normalization
- Bruises, Cuts, Scratches,... Healed Faster
- Cancer (reduced tumors)
- Circulation
- Diabetes (Type Two)
- Dizziness
- Energy Level Increase

- Exercise (longer workouts)
- Glaucomic Eye Pressure
- Hair (restores original color & enhances re-growth)
- High Blood Pressure
- Immune System Enhancement
- Inflammation
- Intestinal & Bowel Maladies
- Lethargic Appetite
- Libido
- Lifespan Increase
- Memory Improvement
- Menopause
- Menstruation
- Mental Clarity
- Migraine Headaches(decrease)
- Morbus Parkinson's Disease
- Nausea
- Pain (general)
- Prostate (PSA)
- Red Blood Cells Live Longer
- Sense of Smell Improvement
- Sense of Taste Improvement
- Sinus Pressure
- Sleep Improvement
- Trembling Hands
- Ulcers (mouth, stomach,...)
- Urinary Maladies
- Vision Improvement
- Weight-Loss

Is Indium safe to take?

Yes. According to tests on animals, the current Indium supplement offered by *East Park Research, Inc.*, it would have to be 1,000 times stronger just to make a mouse sick!

Oh, before I forget, Indium has been given to race horses to improve their performance.

This sounds too good to be true but I'm still very interested in Indium. Where can I get more FREE information before I make my buying decision?

Good question. See *East Park Research, Inc.* in the POC Section.

The Mother Of All Antioxidants: There is something in your body that helps you stay vibrantly healthy and young but this unknown & unique molecule runs low as you age.

And as it runs low, all kinds of bad guys from minor maladies to serious maladies start attacking your body. And physical appearance decline and mental decline surface more and more.

What if you can get some of the youth back in your life? What if you can get more of this SUPER POWERFUL ANTIOXIDANT THAT IS 5,000 TIMES STRONGER THAN OTHER ANTIOXIDANTS!!!

Here it is - it's called GLUTATHIONE! Glutathione is being manufactured in your body right now - this very second.

But its production diminishes as you grow older. Once you reach 60 years of age, your glutathione production is cut in half (50%).

Normal levels of Glutathione provide:
- After-Burner Energy
- Cardiovascular improvement
- Elderly physical appearance reversed
- Fast recall
- Flexible and pain free joints
- Hair regrowth
- Improved digestion
- Improved immune system
- Longevity
- Original hair color
- Powerful detoxifier
- Robust health
- Sharp mental focus
- Vision improvement
- **Weight-Loss**
- And much more

More than **80,000 published scientific studies PROVE** the iron clad guaranteed health benefits of Glutathione.

But what if you could get more of this amazing *Fountain of Youth*? How? Where?

MOST IMPORTANT NOTE: I thought this segment was so important I went out and purchased my own *Glutathione*. I purchased a bottle at GNC called *L- Glutathione (500 mg - 60 capsules)*. It costs $38.65 (02-month supply). On 29 Sep. 2017, I took one capsule with a soda drink.

And no foolin', I felt better in about 45-minutes. I skipped a day and didn't feel as good. On 01 October I took another and I can say there is something to this *Glutathione*. I'll be taking the 02-month supply and plan on seeing what happens.

The Root Of All Sickness: You've heard the saying *"Money Is The Root Of All Evil."* Well after years of research, I'm (author) thinking that *"Sugar Is The Root Of All Sickness."* I'm no scientist, I'm no doctor and I'm no nutritionist. Those professionals are academically 1,000 smarter than I am.

However, I'm just an underpaid survival teacher. Since writing these books:

- *"The Gettysburg Program - What You Don't Know May Be Killing You. Your Complete Guide To Better Health And Vibrant Living!"* (600+ pages)
- *"99+ International Heart Attack Preventers, Fighters, Killers And More!"*
- *"99+ International Cancer Preventers, Cancer Fighters, Cancer Killers And More!"*
- *"99+ International Diabetes Preventers, Fighters, Killers And More!"*

See **www.survivalexpertbooks.com**

I'm convinced of all *The Five Deadly Whites* – in my humble opinion, **SUGAR** is the worst of the worst.
You must read – re-read:
- Carbohydrates Are Slowly Killing You Right Now
- Fructose Is Slowly Killing You Right Now
- Dr. Vernon's Diabetes Remedy
- Eskimo Diabetes Cure
- Foods, Snacks And Drinks With Low & No Carbohydrates
- My Family Stopped Eating Sugar For A Year And This Is What Happened

Train Track Healing Treatment: In West Java, Indonesia, the local people really believe that their ailments can be cured by electricity. And the electricity they use come from railway train tracks. The local people lay in the center of the tracks and reach out with both hands touching the rails to their left and right completing the electrical circuit. Some lay their whole body across both rails insuring the circuit is complete. Does the *Train Track Healing Treatment* really work? Those locals may be on to something. See *Car Jack Headache Cure*.

Tumeric: Tumeric is the main spice (bright yellow color) found in curry powder / curry dishes. But for this segment we'll concentrate on Tumeric. Tumeric has been used in India for its medicinal benefits for thousands of years.

One of tumeric's compounds – curcumin, it alone has a laundry list of healing benefits behind it. It's reported that curcumin may be more beneficial than using a variety of prescription drugs.

Tumeric provides vitamin B6, vitamin C, calcium, copper, iron, manganese, potassium and zinc. But the most valuable is the compound curcumin.

Tumeric has a list of healthy benefits to fight, heal, relieve maladies like:
- Acne
- Alzheimer's Disease
- Antibacterial
- Anti-cancer properties
- Anti-inflammatory
- Antitumor
- Anti-ulcer
- Antiviral
- Arthritis relief
- Brain booster
- Bronchitis
- Burns
- Dandruff
- Detoxes the liver
- Diabetes
- Diarrhea
- Dry skin
- Eczema
- Eliminates intestinal worms

- Facial hair
- Fights foreign invaders
- Hair growth
- Headaches
- Heals wounds
- Heart health
- High blood pressure
- Improves immune system
- Indigestion
- Jaundice
- Liver health
- Lowers bad cholesterol (LDL)
- Menstrual cramps
- Oily skin
- Pain relief
- Pink eye (conjunctivitis)
- Reduces depression
- Scalp treatment
- Skin lightening
- Stretch marks
- Strong antioxidant
- Weight-Loss
- Wrinkles

After conducting my 'intensive research' on Tumeric, I decided to add it on a regular basis to my own updated *Laydon's Healing Spice Concoction*. By the way, back in 1994, I discovered that cayenne pepper (150,000 SHU) CURED my almost 40-years of super painful paralyzing back spasms.

U.S. Army Rifle Drill Exercises (07): If you want to tone-up and get in-shape, here are 07 Rifle Drill. These Rifle Drill Exercises will **surprise you at their effectiveness**. The 1st time you try them, I guarantee you'll be sore the next morning.

These Rifle Drills were used during <u>Phase 01</u> of the U.S. Army Special Forces Qualification Course (Green Berets) - early 1980s, for they gave the Special Forces candidate a great muscle strengthening workout. Anyway, while teaching SROTC at Mercer University in Macon, Georgia - early 1990s, every once in a while, I had to discipline a cadet here and there.

And the way I did it was with some extra PT (physical training). One day I had these 04 MS IIIs (Juniors) who needed such discipline so I had them assemble in the large dayroom where the cadets formed-up for formation.

I taught the 04 cadets the 06 Rifle Drills and assigned each cadet a specific rifle drill to learn and copycat so they could each take their turns in repeating the Rifle Drills.

The Rifle Drill were conducted with a **<u>07-pound</u>** rubber weapon that looks just like an M16 assault rifle. I taught all 06 Rifle Drills with 15 repetitions of each Rifle Drill - a good warm-up. Then each cadet took their own turn on their respective Rifle Drill and exercised the other 03 cadets.

Instead of 15 repetitions, they each did 25 repetitions of each Rifle Drill. So now that's a total of 40 repetitions they exercised on each Rifle Drill. The next morning the cadets woke-up in their own rooms and were extremely sore. So sore they hurt all over their bodies. I just chuckled when I heard of their conditions.

Now each Rifle Drill has either a 04-count (movement) or 08 count (movement) to it. And each Rifle Drill is also done at a slow pace, moderate pace or a fast pace. The following are instructions for each Rifle Drill and their sketches straight out of the Army's training manual FM 21-20 Physical Fitness Training.

Note: No you don't have to have a 07-pound M16 weapon to negotiate the Rifle Drills. You can use other items that are thin, approximately 36-inches long and weighs approximately 07-pounds, 06-pounds, or less if you prefer.

Rifle Drill Counting Of Each Movement And Repetition!

Now to properly count each repetition, count each 04-count movement for example like 1, 2, 3, **1**; 1, 2, 3, **2**; 1, 2, 3, **3**; 1, 2, 3, **4**; 1, 2, 3, **5**;...

And count each 08-count exercise like 1, 2, 3, 4, 5, 6, 7, **1**; 1, 2, 3, 4, 5, 6, 7, **2**; 1, 2, 3, 4, 5, 6, 7, **3**; 1, 2, 3, 4, 5, 6, 7, **4**;... And remember to adhere to the cadence for each exercise whether it's slow, moderate or fast pace.

Do at least 15 repetitions of each exercise and you'll get a great workout. Don't have a 07-pound M16? No big deal. Improvise, just make sure the exercise tool you use is at least 07-pounds for a worthy workout. Yes you can use a 06-pound, 05-pound,... workout tool.

OK, let's start with the 1st US Army Rifle Drill – the *Fore-Up, Behind Back*.

Try to start out with 15 Repetitions of each the 06 Rifle Drills and finish up with the 7th Rifle Drill Exercise and work up from there.

May be one day I'll produce a video for the *U.S. Army Rifle Drill Exercises (07).*

Rifle Drill #01
Fore-Up, Behind Back!

This is a four count exercise done at a moderate cadence.

The starting position, hold the rifle downward and feet together.

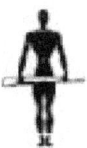

Swing arms forward and upward to overhead position.

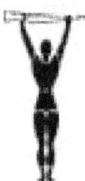

Lower rifle to back of shoulders.

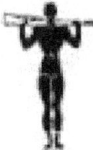

Move to first position.

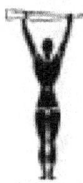

Recover to starting position.

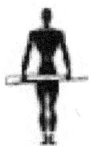

Rifle Drill #02
Fore-Up, Back Bend!

This is a four-count exercise done at a moderate cadence.

The starting position, hold rifle downward and feet together.

Swing arms forward and up to overhead position.

Bend backward, emphasizing bend in upper back. Keep face up and knees straight.

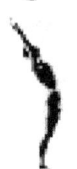

Move to first position.

Recover to start position.

Rifle Drill #03
Up And Forward!

This is a four-count exercise done at a fast cadence.

To starting position, hold rifle downward and feet together.

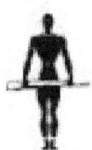

Swing arms forward and upward to overhead position.

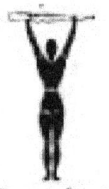

Swing arms forward to shoulder level.

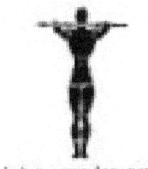

Move to first position.

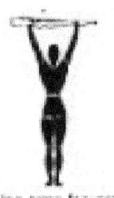

Recover to start position.

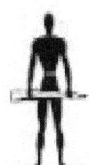

Rifle Drill #04
Fore-Up, Squat!

This is a four-count exercise done at a moderate cadence.
The starting position, hold rifle downward and feet approximately shoulder
width apart.

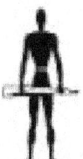

Swing arms forward and upward to overhead position.

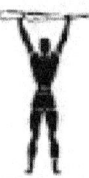

Swing arms down to shoulder level and assume a half-knee-bend position.

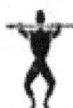

Move to first position.

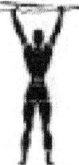

Recover to start position.

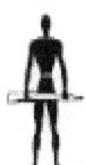

Rifle Drill #05
Fore-Up, Side Bend!

This is a four-count exercise done at a slow cadence.

The starting position, hold the rifle in front of you at eye-level with both arms locked in the horizontal position.

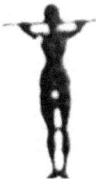

Bend the upper body to the left while keeping the arms horizontally locked and holding the weapon.

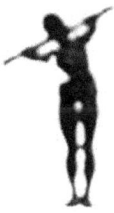

Return to the 1st position.

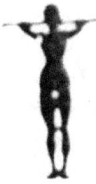

Bend the upper body to the right while keeping the arms horizontally locked and holding the weapon.

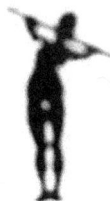

Return to the 1st position.

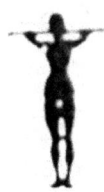

Rifle Drill #06
Fore-Up, Lunger!

This is a 08-count exercise done a moderate cadence.

The starting position, hold rifle downward and feet together.

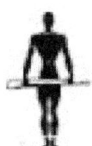

Step to the half-left with the left foot. At the same time, raise the weapon straight above the head with the arms locked vertically.

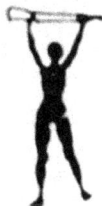

Bend downward keeping the arms locked and swinging the weapon downward so it's finally positioned outside the left ankle.

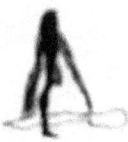

Straighten-up bringing the weapon straight above the head with the arms locked vertically.

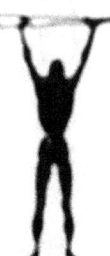

Return to the starting position.

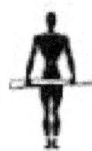

Step to the half-right with the right foot. At the same time, raise the weapon straight above the
head with the arms locked vertically.

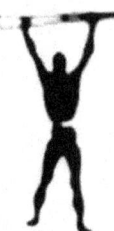

Bend downward keeping the arms locked and swinging the weapon downward so it's finally positioned outside the right ankle.

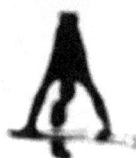

Straighten-up bringing the weapon straight above the head with the arms locked vertically.

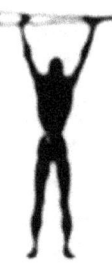

Return to the starting position.

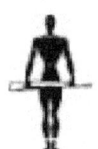

Rifle Drill #07
Horizontal Hold!

This static exercise should be done after completing all 06 Rifle Drills. It will hurt but it builds stamina and strength. Place feet shoulder width apart and your body erect. Raise your weapon up in front of you at eye level with your arms and the weapon in a *"stiff"* horizontal position. Insure elbows are locked.

Now hold the weapon in this position for a full 03-minutes. Each day you workout, add a little more time each time you do this last exercise. Yes, you'll feel the BURN but you're burning calories!!!!

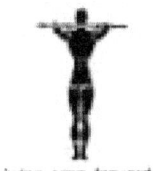

IMPORTANT NOTE: Check with your doctor before negotiating the *07 U.S Army Rifle Drills*.

See *Jail House Workout.*

Visualizations Done By Saints: Folks as you know, I've talked about the POWERS of visualization and I've talked about it throughout my writing career. Here's another "angle" on Visualization.

Throughout history, there's evidence that Saints have used Visualization. Saints and those "chosen ones" have seen Visualizations in broad daylight where others see nothing!

Even today throughout the US and the world, ordinary folks see Visualizations where the person next to them see nothing! Those Visualizations have CHANGED the visualizee for the better.

One particular Saint I want to talk about is ***Saint Peregrine - Patron Saint For Cancer Patients***. Let me give you the story on this Saint.

Saint Peregrine was born in 1256 in Forli, Italy. Not much data is known in his early days. But as an adult, Peregrine was recorded to have attacked a peacemaker sent by the Pope.

Forli was governed by the Pope and Peregrine was actively involved in anti-papal activities. Forli was restricted from celebrating the Mass and Sacraments. At a town meeting, was when Peregrine attacked the peacemaker sent by the Pope - Servitude Superior General, Saint Philip Benizi.

Saint Benizi advised Peregrine to seek guidance from Our Lady of Sorrows. Peregrine channelized his energies into caring good works and at the age of 30, he joined the Servants of Mary, Servite Order. Peregrine eventually returned to Forli and devoted his life of caring for the sick and hopeless.

Peregrine in an act of penance for himself, stood instead of sitting every chance he could. This led to varicose veins which deteriorated into an open sore on one if his legs. The sore was diagnosed as cancer. The open sore was so odorous and painful, Peregrine's surgeon strongly advised amputation.

Visualization Of Christ!

Peregrine agreed and the night before the surgery, Peregrine prayed. He prayed using a Visualization of Christ on the Cross.

His deep prayers put him in a trance and ***"he envisioned the crucified Christ leaving the cross and touching his cancerous leg."*** The very next morning, Peregrine was completely cured.

On 01 May 1344, at the age of 80, Peregrine died. He was later canonized (became an official Saint) on 27 December, 1726 and is known as the Patron Saint for those who suffer from cancer. His feast day is on 04 May each year.

Now there's NOTHING WRONG with **copy-catting Saint Peregrine's same visualization** of seeing Christ leave the cross and touching the maladies in your body.

The following is the official prayer to Saint Peregrine. Remember what I told you about Prayer - it's one of the most POWERFUL Mind-Over-Matter Applications.

Prayer To Saint Peregrine

Dear Saint Peregrine, they need your help. They feel so uncertain of their lives right now. This serious illness makes them long for a sign of God's love. Help them to imitate your enduring faith when you faced the ugliness of cancer and surgery. Allow them to trust the Lord the way you did in the moment of distress.

They want to be cured, but right now they ask God for strength to bear this cross in their lives. They seek the power to proclaim God's presence in their lives despite the hardship, anguish, and fear they now experience. O Glorious Saint Peregrine, be an inspiration to them and petitioner of these needed graces from our loving Father. Amen.

O God, who gave to saint Peregrine an Angel for his companion, the Mother of God for his teacher, and Jesus for the Physician of his malady; grant, we pray that through his merits, we may on Earth intensely love our Holy Angel, the Blessed Virgin, and Our savior, and in Heaven bless them forever. Grant that we may receive the favor for which we now petition, FOR ALL THOSE SUFFERING FROM CANCER OR OTHER LIFE-THREATENING DISEASES. Through the same Christ our Lord. Amen.
Follow with an Our Father, Hail Mary, and Glory Be.

WHEAT GERM WEIGHT-LOSS: Wheat germ is part of the wheat plant that's responsible for sprouting and making new wheat plants. The wheat germ is <u>alive with life</u> and is made-up of proteins, vitamins and minerals.

Anyway, quite some time back, I interviewed a friend who told me their mother lost weight using wheat germ. All she did was add wheat germ to EVERYTHING she ate.

From breakfast to dinner meals and even snacks, wheat germ was always part of the meal. It was as simple as that. I use Kretschmer Wheat Germ. It's an excellent healthy food additive.

Note: Try a hefty combination of Wheat Germ (03 tablespoons), Sprouts (02 handfuls) and your favorite salad dressing for a super healthy meal. See *Wheat Germ Oil For After-Burner Performance* right below and see *Sprouts*.

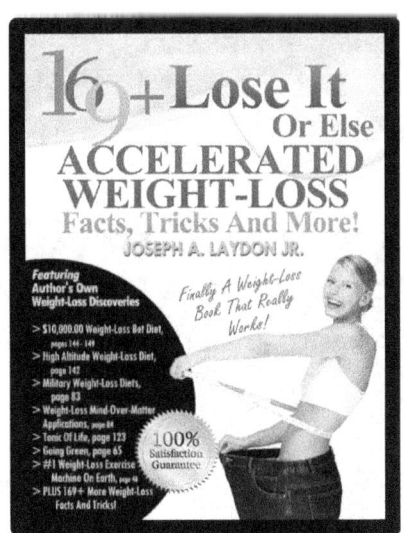

Search For This Book At

www.amazon.com

WHEAT GERM OIL FOR AFTER-BURNER PERFORMANCE: Here's a health supplement worthy of your attention and it may give you that after-burner performance. This healthy supplement is called wheat germ oil. Again, wheat germ is part of the wheat plant that's responsible for sprouting and making new wheat plants.

The wheat germ is <u>alive with life</u> and is made-up of proteins, vitamins and minerals. Just a half-cup of wheat germ contains 24 grams of protein. It includes minerals like calcium, copper, manganese, magnesium and potassium. It also includes B Vitamins and Vitamin E.

Now wheat germ oil is pressed out of the wheat germ. The wheat germ oil is rich in fat soluble Vitamins. According to Dr. T. K. Cureton, head of the University of Illinois Physical Fitness Laboratory, wheat germ oil may help maintain endurance in athletic performance.

A single daily teaspoon of wheat germ oil along with exercise has shown **to increase men's physical endurance by as much as a whopping 51%!** This amazing find was based on Dr. Cureton's 04-year research that includes tests on 200 men including college men, middle-aged men, swimmers, wrestlers,...

According to Dr. Cureton, *"Wheat germ oil is a valuable dietary supplement to men doing hard exercise and it has possible application to competitive sports. We have tried it sufficiently to believe that this is true.*

It provides something that enables men to bear hard stress and continue to do hard labor without deteriorating. It particularly affects physical endurance and heart response."

Note: All the B Vitamins aid to maintain healthy eyes, hair, liver, mouth, muscle tone in the gastrointestinal tract, nerves and skin. B-Complex Vitamins are coenzymes involved in energy production. B-Complex Vitamins may be useful to **combat depression or anxiety**. The B Vitamins should be taken together.

VPJ Inventor – Robert Augustus Chesebrough!

In 1859, chemist Robert Augustus Chesebrough of Brooklyn, New York invented petroleum jelly. That year, Chesebrough travelled to Titusville, Pennsylvania to enter the petroleum oil business but fate brought him to discover the uses of a residue that stuck and clogged drilling parts, pumps,... that had oil workers cussing up a storm.

It turns out oil workers used the sticky dark waste product to help heal wounds, burns,... it accelerated healing. Chesebrough returned to Brooklyn with jars of the petroleum waste product and after months of R&D (Research & Development), Chesebrough extracted the clear essential ingredient(s) and called it *"petroleum jelly."*

To test his petroleum jelly as a healing ingredient, Chesebrough inflicted wounds of burns, cuts, scratches,... on his person and applied petroleum jelly.

To his satisfaction all his wounds healed without a hint of infection. **By 1870, Chesebrough was manufacturing the 1st *Vaseline Petroleum Jelly* (VPJ)**. And over the last 148-years, here are some of the survival uses of *Vaseline Petroleum Jelly* (VPJ).

VPJ Chesebrough Healer: Chesebrough swore by VPJ (*Vaseline Petroleum Jelly*) as a healer. He actually swallowed a spoonful of it each day. In his late 50s, Chesebrough came down with sickly pleurisy (inflammation of the sac near lungs causing coughing, trouble breathing,...). Chesebrough ordered his nurse to give him a spoonful of VPJ and sure enough, his health improved. **CHESEBROUGH CARRIED-ON WITH HIS DAILY REGIMEN OF VPJ AND LIVED ANOTHER 40-YEARS MORE** till he passed away in 1933.

White Sugar Cure: Now in case that burn wound turned infectious here's a long lost remedy used long ago and can still be used today in emergency situations for minor wounds (burns, cuts, diabetic wounds, scrapes,...). It's white refined sugar.

Now I'm not sure exactly how and why it works but white refined sugar was used to heal infectious wounds long before conventional medicine was established. White refined sugar is simply placed at the wound site and wrapped with clean bandages when needed. There are cases where this application even reversed gangrene.

Points Of Contact

Important Note: The following POCs could change their address and phone number or go out of business at any time.

Alternatives- Mountain
Home Publishing---------------1-800-527-3044
Alternatives- Mountain Home Publishing, P.O. Box 2000, Ranson, WV 25438-2000. Alternatives- Mountain Home Publishing offers REAL alternatives to remedy sickly and deadly conditions versus expensive conventional drugs and surgery. Alternatives- Mountain Home Publishing offers a bounty of healthy information. Get their FREE 50-page booklet before you buy.

American Board of
Chelation Therapy, The--------1-312-787-2228
The American Board of Chelation Therapy, 70 W. Huron Street, Chicago, IL 60610. There are over 150 doctors in the U.S. who are certified by the American Board of Chelation Therapy as approved Chelation Therapist. Contact the organization above for a Certified Chelation Therapist in your area. See *Chelation Therapy* in the POC Section.

American College of
Advancement in Medicine, The--1-800-532-3688
                              1-714-583-7666
The American College of Advancement in Medicine (ACAM), 23121 Verdugo Drive, Suite 204, Laguna Hills, CA 92653. A group of more than *600 physicians who put patients first* by using therapies noted to be beneficial.

If you suffer from Alzheimer's disease, arthritis, scleroderma or Raynaud's phenomenon, contact ACAM for a referral. There are also over 150 doctors in the U.S. who are certified by the American Board of Chelation Therapy as approved Chelation Therapist.

Contact the organization above for a certified Chelation Therapist in your area. You may *obtain a list* of ACAM physicians in your area by sending a large SASE to Stanley Jacob, M.D., L225 Oregon Health Sciences University, Portland, OR 97201. See American Preventive Medical Association and American Board of Chelation Therapy in this section.

Association for Research Enlightenment, Inc. (ARE)-----1-800-333-4499
                              1-804-428-3588
                              1-804-422-4631(fax)

Association for Research Enlightenment, Inc., (ARE) continues the work of a man named Edgar Cayce who founded the ARE in 1931. ARE is an international network of people and volunteers who are interested ancient civilizations, dream interpretation, ESP & psychic development, holistic healing, meditation, reincarnation, spiritual growth, the purpose of life, and much more.

There are many benefits to ARE members such as: ARE Camp, ARE Conferences and Seminars, ARE books by mail, The *New Millennium Journal*, *Venture Inward* Magazine, and much more. They'll send you a catalog of their books. One of which is called *The Oil That Heals*(Castor Oil). Call Monday through Friday from 8:00 a.m. to 5:00 p.m., Eastern Standard Time, for your FREE information packet! Offers a very informative book that reveals the healing benefits of castor oil - it's called *The Oil That Heals* by William A. Mc Garey, M.D.!**

Biogenetics Inc.--------------**1-800-630-7789**
Biogenetics, Inc., 101 North Euclid, Bradley, IL 60915.
Biogenetics, Inc. offers a product called FLEXAGENE.
FLEXAGENE is reported to restore flexibility of backs,
elbows, fingers, hips, knees, necks, shoulders,... and
alleviate pain, stiffness, swelling,... FLEXAGENE
helps joints lacking in cartilage regenerate new
cartilage and synovial fluids (joint lubrication).

At the age of 40, cartilage loss is as much as 40%. By
the age of 50, cartilage loss can be as high as 60%.
By the age of 60, cartilage loss could be as high as
75%. Simple activities like bending, dancing, dressing
yourself, sewing, shaving, walking,... could be a
fight, a painful fight. FLEXAGENE is reported to
outperform and is safer than celebrex, cortisone,
glucosomine, ibuprofen, steroids, and vioxx. Before
you purchase anything, call or write for their FREE 12-
page, all-color brochure.

Note: Biogenetics Inc., also offers another painful
joint remedy called *OPC Miracle Joint Complex*.

Chelation Therapy-------------see **American Board of
Chelation Therapy, The**.

Concord Grape Juice----------**www.concordgrapejuice.com**

**Country Doctor's Big Bag
Of Common Sense Cures, The----unavailable**
Health Revelations, Order Processing Center, P.O. Box
925, Frederick, MD 21705-9913.

```
----------------Crystal Healing POCs----------------

Aumara Light &
Healing Circle, The----------www.aumara.com

Cavern Crystals----------------www.crystalcavern.com

Crystal And
Healing Federation-----------www.crystalandhealing.com

Crystal Healing Center-----www.crystalhealingcenter.com

Crystal Links----------------www.crystalinks.com

Healing Music
Organization, The------------www.healingmusic.org
----------------End Of Crystal Healing POCs------------
```

**Discovering The
Power Of Self-Hypnosis--------by Stanley Fisher, Ph.D.**

East Park Research, Inc.------1-888-374-2363
East Park Research, Inc., 2709 Horseshoe Drive, Las Vegas, NV 89120-3337. Call or write East Park research, Inc., and ask to be put on their mailing list. In particular, ask for their 96-page booklet *Indium - The Missing Trace Mineral*, written by Dr. Robert Lyons. Once you receive their material, decide if Indium is for you then see your doctor for a final go-ahead.

Graviola And How It Can Heal The Cancer (the secret of graviola fruit and how it can kill cancer cells: 10000 times stronger killer of cancer than chemotherapy)--------------------by GyoBy Brand

Healthy Living----------------1-800-800-0100
www.amerimark.com   1-440-826-1267(fax)
Healthy Living, 6836 Engle Road, P.O. Box 94512, Cleveland, OH 44101-4512. Healthy Living offers hundreds of products you have to at least take a look at by browsing through their 56-page, all-color catalog. They offer hundreds of products from gadgets to health products to make your life more comfortable. I've received a few thousand catalogs from a hundred or so companies, that offer a kazillion products over the years and Healthy Living has many products I've never seen before. Call or write today for your own catalog. And yes, if you hurry, they offer FREE shipping (as of Summer 2003).

Heintzman Farms---------------1-888-333-5813
Heintzman Farms, Rural Route 2 Box 265, Onaka, SD 57466. Mr. Rick Heintzman owner of Heintzman Farms offers a kit that includes three 01-pound bags of Dakota Gold flax seed, an electric grinder and two home cholesterol test kits for only $70. If you want a free sample of flax seeds send a SASE! Heintzman Farms also offers 01-pound bags of flax seed or in bulk.

HomeHealth-Solutions
For Healthy Living------------1-800-284-9123
HomeHealth, 3890 Park Central Blvd. North, Pompano Beach, FL 33064. HomeHealth is the "Official Supplier of Edgar Cayce Products." Home Health offers hundreds of healthy products like Castor Oil and Wool Flannel Sheets. Other products are too numerous to mention.

Their 40-page catalog is packed with super healthy products and even products for kittie and bowser! Call for your FREE all-color catalog today!**

Home Remedies That Work-------by Joan Wilen.

Hypnotize Yourself
Out Of Pain Now!-------------by Bruce N. Eimer,
                         Ph.D., ABPP

Institute for Vibrant Health--1-800-218-1379
Institute for Vibrant Health, 4525 Purple Sage Trail, Cottonwood, AZ 86326. Institute for Vibrant Health offers an exercise machine just for the super healthy benefits of rebound exercise. For more information on this healthy exercise, call or write for their free 16-page, all-color brochure.

-----------------Jerry Baker POCs---------------
Amazing Antidotes------------www.jerrybaker.com

Back To Nature Almanac #1-----www.jerrybaker.com

Backyard Problem Solver Book--www.jerrybaker.com

Critter Control &
Pest Prevention---------------www.jerrybaker.com

Flower Power------------------www.jerrbaker.com

Giant Book Of Garden Secrets--www.jerrybaker.com

Great Green Book Of
Garden Secrets---------------www.jerrybaker.com

Green Grass Magic------------www.jerrybaker.com

Happy Healthy Houseplants-----www.jerrybaker.com

Impatient Gardener, The-------www.jerrybaker.com

Impatient Gardener
Lawnbook, The-----------------www.jerrybaker.com

Jerry Bakers Lawn Book--------www.jerrybaker.com

Kitchen Counter Cures--------www.jerrybaker.com

Old Time Gardening Wisdom-----www.jerrybaker.com

Secrets - Test Gardens--------www.jerrybaker.com

Talk To Your Plants----------www.jerrybaker.com

Note: If not available, E-Bay may have what you need.
----------------**End Of Jerry Baker POCs**----------

Luke Chan--------------------**www.chilel.com**
101 Miracles of Natural Healing at www.amazon.com

YouTube------------Natural Healing - Chi Lel Qigong
Back in the late 1990s, I talked to Luke Chan and he surprised me that he was a down to Earth person. Very helpful. I was doing my research on alternative health practices and called his office and was surprised when he answered the phone.

Miraculous Health - How To
Heal Your Body By Unleashing
The Hidden Power Of Your Mind-by Dr. Rick Levy

Natural Medicine Associates
Customer Service--------------1-800-408-1525
                Order Line---1-800-388-7012
Natural Medicine Associates, 4094 Majestic Lane,Suite 107, Fairfax, VA 22033. Natural Medicine Associates offers the "Total Body Cleanse" for colon build-up and several parasites that cause or are linked to many afflictions. Like acne, allergies, cancer, constipation, diarrhea, bloating, chronic fatigue, granulomas, irritable bowel syndrome, joint pains, muscle pains, overweight, nervousness, skin conditions, sleep disturbances, tooth grinding...

According to Natural Medicine Associates, *"the average person over 40 has anywhere between 5 to 25 pounds of build-up in their colons..."* Colon build up is a serious and unknown health problem and so are the many parasites found in humans. Parasites like the beef worm, female roundworm, hook worm, liver fluke, pin worm, schistosome fluke, three-lip ascaris, whole worm...!

Don't believe me, go to the Internet and type in "parasite" you'll browse and eventually get some real shocking pictures of these parasites that are robbing you of your health! Look into a "total body cleanse" and call or write for FREE information today - get on their mailing list!!!

Nutrition Coalition, Inc.-----1-800-447-4793
www.willardswater.com   1-218-236-9783
**   1-218-236-6753(fax)**
Nutrition Coalition, Inc., P.O. Box 3001, Fargo, ND 58108-3001. Nutrition Coalition, Inc. offers an authentic **<u>Willard Water</u>**. Remember, the healing sneaks up on you so write down all maladies before consumption!

Powers Of Healing-------------Time - Life Books

-----Prickly Pear Cactus Products POCs------
Prepair----------------------1-800-720-2970
Offers prickly pear capsules called Prepair.

Prickly Pear Cactus Juice-----1-800-205-9499
www.juniperridge.com
-------End Of Prickly Pear Cactus Products POCs---

The Country Doctor's Big Bag Of Common Sense Cures

Special Cancer Fighting / Cancer Killer Videos And More!

Cancer Cure - Baking Soda
And Molasses (00:04:13)--------------------YouTube

Cancer Disappears With Water
Fasting - Dr. Alan Goldhamer (00:03:33)----YouTube

Fasting Kills Cancer (00:07:02)------------YouTube

Water Fasting Kills
Cancer Cells (00:04:05)--------------------YouTube

Vitamin Shoppe----------------1-800-223-1216
www.vitaminshoppe.com   1-800-852-7153**(fax)**
Vitamin Shoppe, The, 4700 Westside Avenue, North
Bergen, New Jersey 07047. The Vitamin Shoppe offers a
large selection (over 14,000 items in stock) of
Vitamins, herbs and homeopathic remedies. "Compare and
Save! 20% to 40% Off Nationally Advertised Brands."

Call or write to get their latest seasonal all color,
100-page catalog. Vitamin Shoppe's catalog is very
informative. You'll learn by simply browsing through
their pages eye-catching and healthy products.

More Survival Kindle E-Books And Survival Paperback Books For YOU!

Joseph A. Laydon Jr. (MSG Ret. Army) is the author and owner of Intensive Research Information Services And Products (IRISAP). Joseph has been writing *"self-reliance"* orientated data since 1991 and since July 2012 has been re-publishing his works via Kindle E-Books and CreateSpace Paperback Books. He has self-published more than **90+ Survival Books** (Kindle E-Books and Paperback Books). Below is a partial list of all his Survival Books and you can see these books by simply going to the 02 websites listed below for detailed descriptions and videos. See *"About The Author."*

- **Kindle E-Books:**--------------------**www.survivalexpertebooks.com**

- **Paperback Books:**-----------------**www.survivalexpertbooks.com**

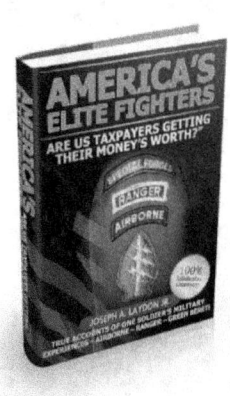 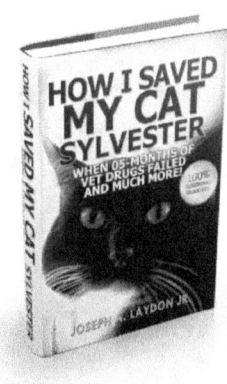 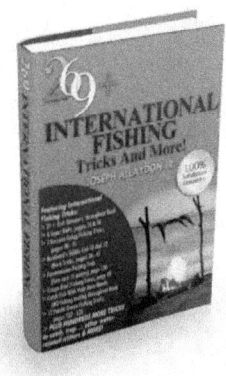

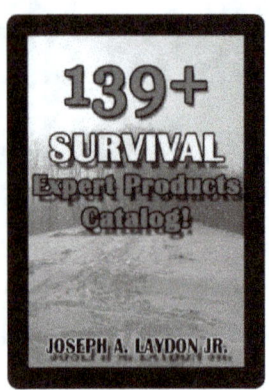

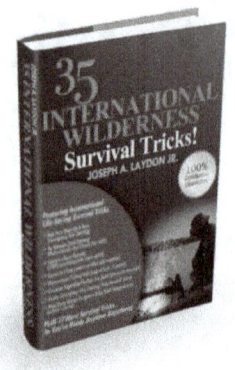

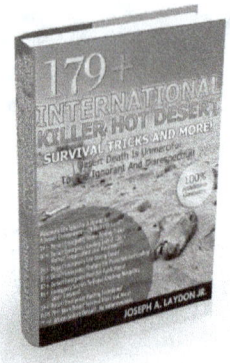

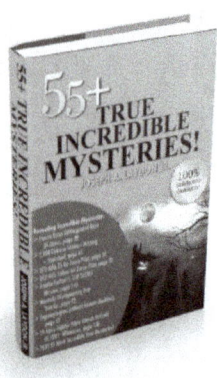

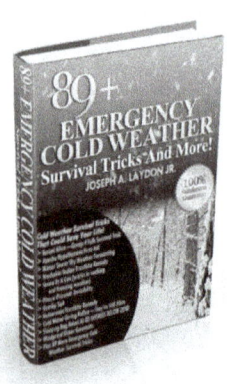

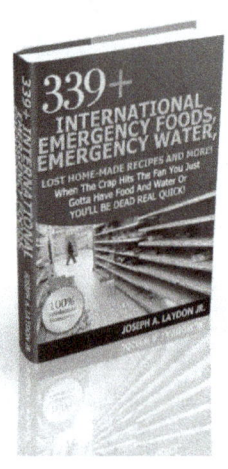

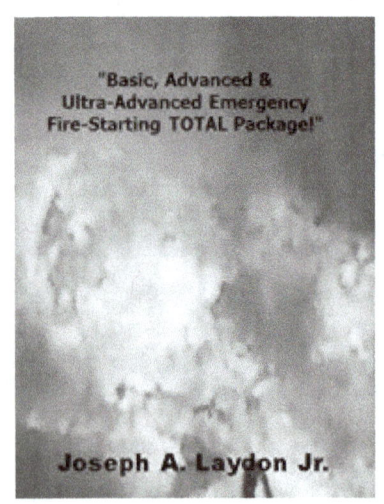

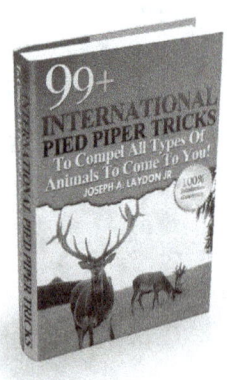

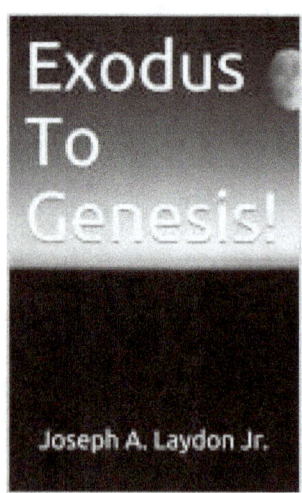

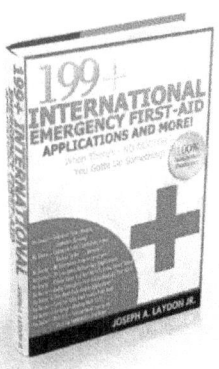
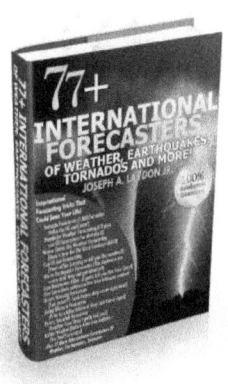
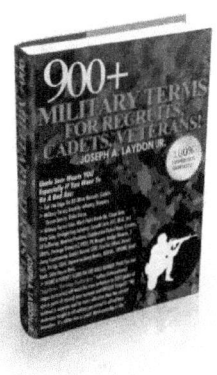

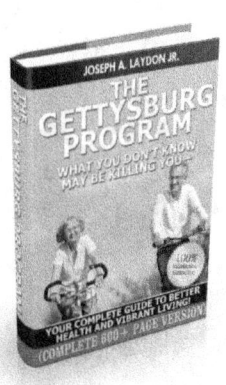
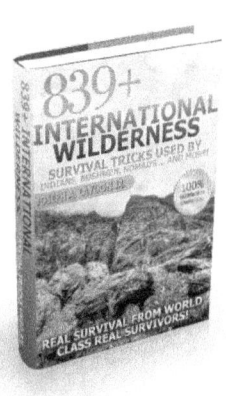
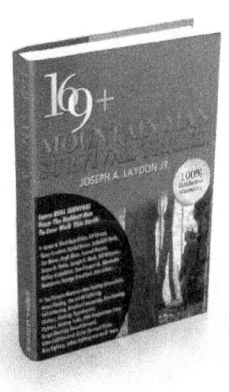

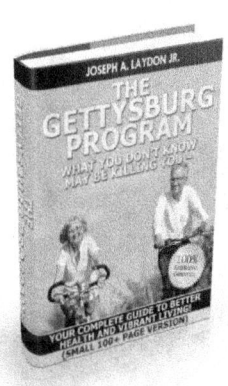
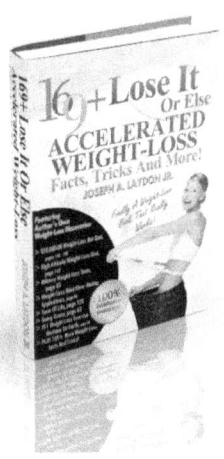
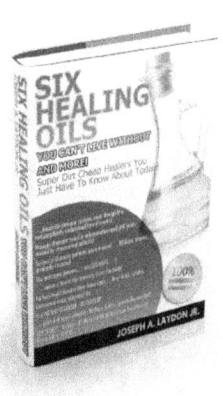

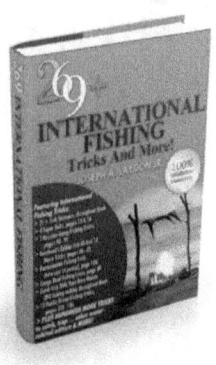

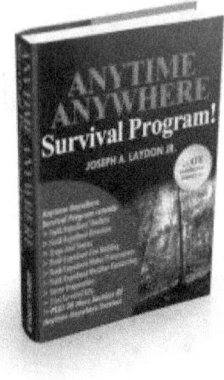

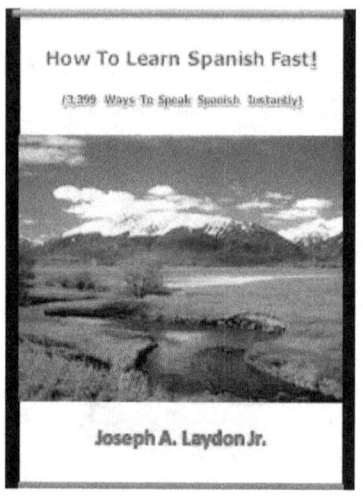

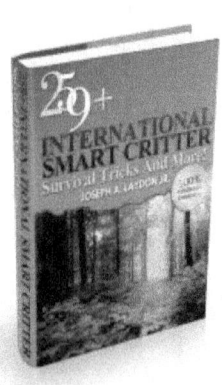

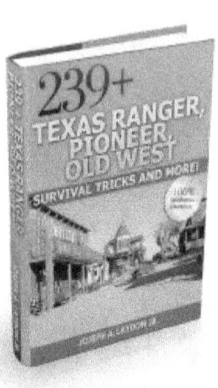

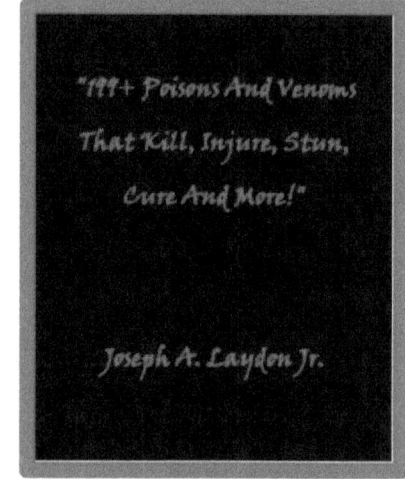

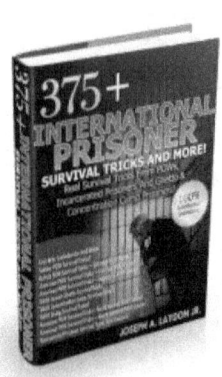

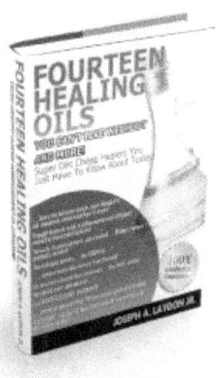

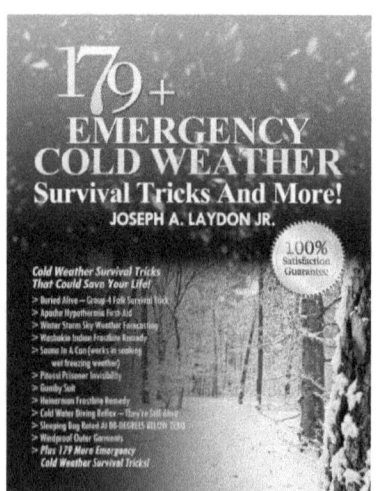

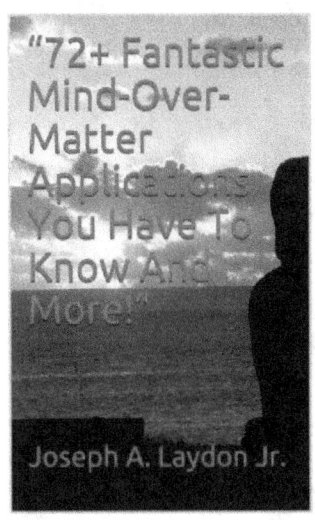

"72+ Fantastic Mind-Over-Matter Applications You Have To Know And More!"

Joseph A. Laydon Jr.

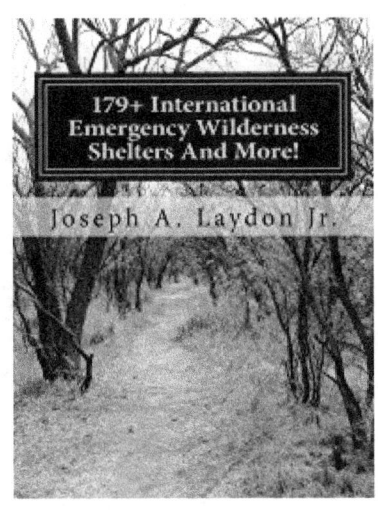

179+ International Emergency Wilderness Shelters And More!

Joseph A. Laydon Jr.

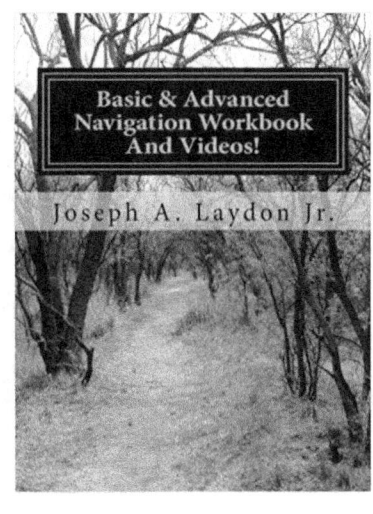

Basic & Advanced Navigation Workbook And Videos!

Joseph A. Laydon Jr.

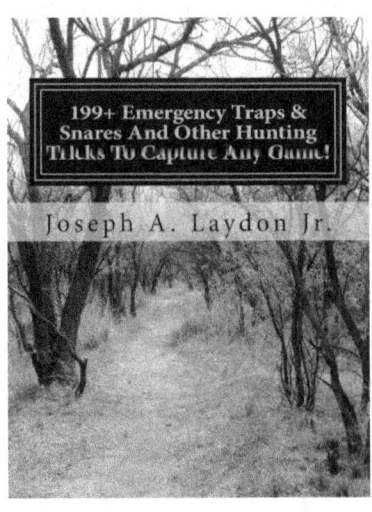

199+ Emergency Traps & Snares And Other Hunting Tricks To Capture Any Game!

Joseph A. Laydon Jr.

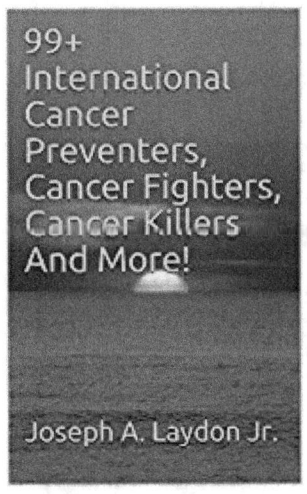

99+ International Cancer Preventers, Cancer Fighters, Cancer Killers And More!

Joseph A. Laydon Jr.

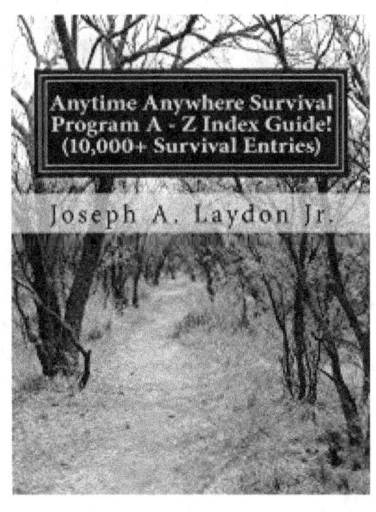

Anytime Anywhere Survival Program A - Z Index Guide! (10,000+ Survival Entries)

Joseph A. Laydon Jr.

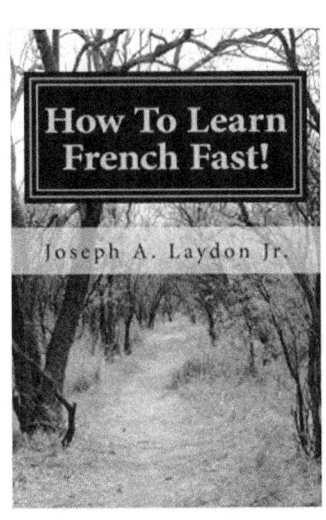

How To Learn French Fast!

Joseph A. Laydon Jr.

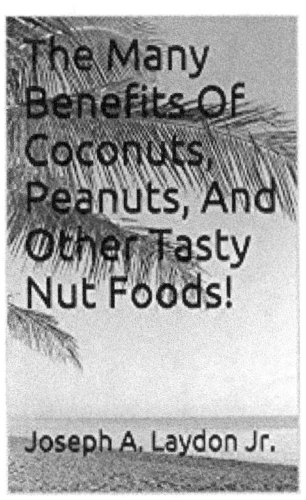

The Many Benefits Of Coconuts, Peanuts, And Other Tasty Nut Foods!

Joseph A. Laydon Jr.

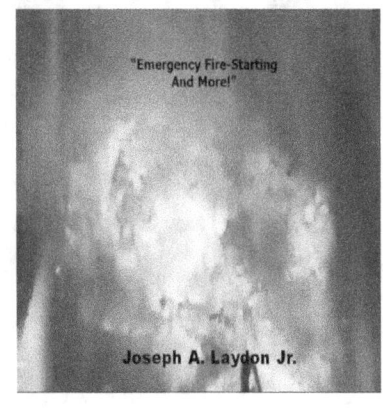

"Emergency Fire-Starting And More!"

Joseph A. Laydon Jr.

213

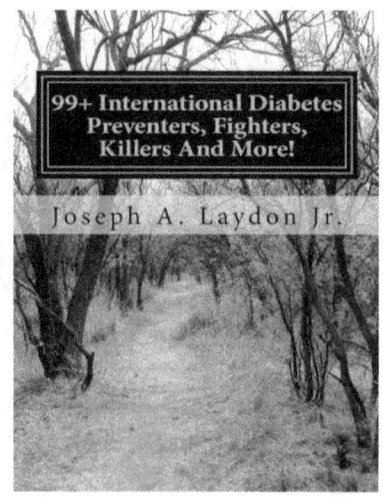

99+ International Diabetes Preventers, Fighters, Killers And More!
Joseph A. Laydon Jr.

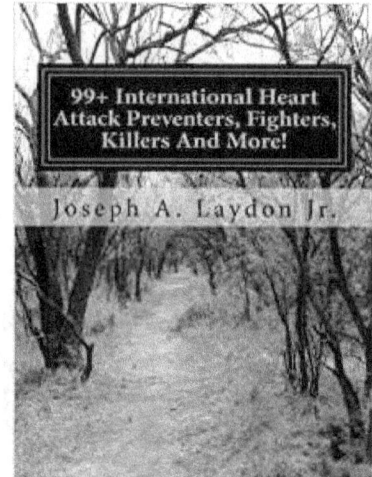

99+ International Heart Attack Preventers, Fighters, Killers And More!
Joseph A. Laydon Jr.

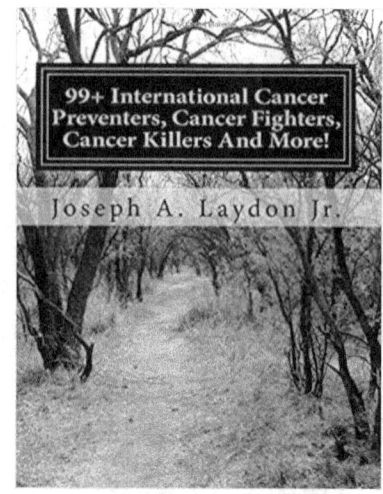

99+ International Cancer Preventers, Cancer Fighters, Cancer Killers And More!
Joseph A. Laydon Jr.

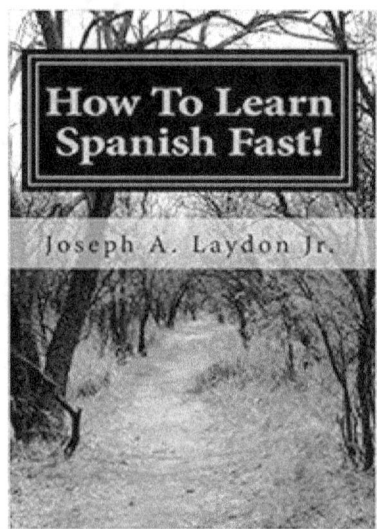

How To Learn Spanish Fast!
Joseph A. Laydon Jr.

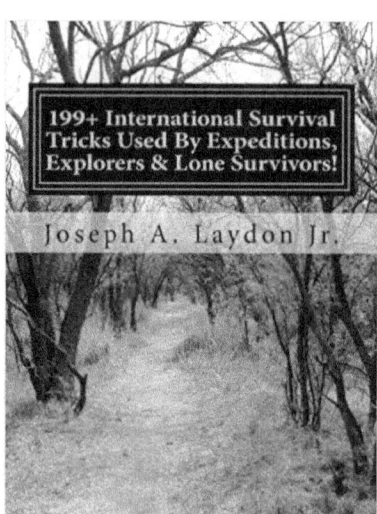

199+ International Survival Tricks Used By Expeditions, Explorers & Lone Survivors!
Joseph A. Laydon Jr.

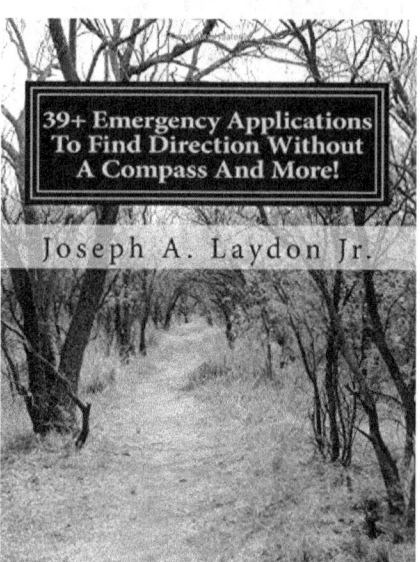

39+ Emergency Applications To Find Direction Without A Compass And More!
Joseph A. Laydon Jr.

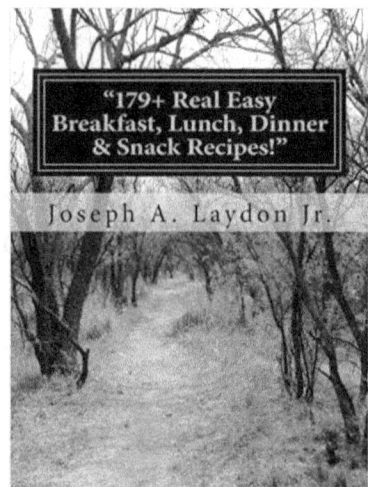

"179+ Real Easy Breakfast, Lunch, Dinner & Snack Recipes!"
Joseph A. Laydon Jr.

About The Author

Joseph A. Laydon Jr. (MSG (E-8) Retired United States Army - 18Z5V) is 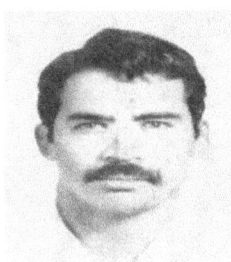 the author and owner of *Intensive Research Information Services And Products (IRISAP)*. Joseph is a well-qualified instructor in international wilderness survival and the other 03 Survivals he teaches (Health Survival, Crime Survival and Money Survival). He is a 20-year US Army veteran (Master Sergeant E-8 - 18Z5V) associated with all Special Operations units in the US military, as well as Special Ops units in the Mid-East and Central & South America.

He's a qualified SERE Instructor (Survival Evasion Resistance & Escape) and has **taught wilderness survival** at the college level for 03 years. He's a qualified instructor in basic & advanced pistol marksmanship, basic & advanced rifle marksmanship, CQB (Close Quarter Battle), basic & advanced cross-country navigation, basic mountaineering techniques, and self-defense. Since 1994, he's published many self-improvement Survival Programs, Survival Videos, SPECIAL Reports, Intelligence Reports, monthly Newsletters, **90+ Survival Books** (Kindle E-Books & CreateSpace Paperback Books) and more in the works.

He's an inventor, he *"sideways engineers"* new survival tricks that can SAVE YOUR LIFE! An example: On 17 August 2000 - 1417 hours, at Scott Lake, Scott AFB, IL, Joseph made international history! He is the 1st in the world to replicate the mysterious fires of Africa using a single drop of water! On 05 January 2001, he discovered how to start a life-saving fire in just 02-seconds using a beam of light from a flashlight in pitch black *"blind man"* darkness! On 06 April 2005 - 1810 hours, he invented delicious & tasty Solid Fuel Rolls and several Trail-Mix Cookies that are used as emergency foods and used as long-burning emergency fire-starting kindling.

And recently - **50+ MORE TOP SECRET INVENTIONS** of advanced & **ultra-advanced fire-starting** like starting EMERGENCY FIRE-STARTING using personal care products and first-aid products you already use like:

- Shampoo

- Toothpastes
- Mouthwashes
- Breath Drops & Breath Sprays
- Salves
- Ointments
- Over-The-Counter Medicines
- Drink Enhancement Products
- Other ingredients like your spit (saliva), your urination,...

See **www.survivalexpert.com/fire**

He also teaches Advanced Navigation (*Basic & Advanced Navigation Workbook And Videos* [includes Workbook, Videos, maps, protractors,…]) so you're ready Anytime Anywhere! Only from IRISAP and only for privileged IRISAP subscribers - YOU! See *Basic & Advanced Navigation Workbook And Videos* at **www.survivalexpertbooks.com/navigation**

Below is a sample of his military achievements & qualifications (**<u>not in chronological order</u>**) which reflect his unique & superior ability to teach basic, advanced & ultra-advanced survival applications, techniques and "tricks" that could help you AVOID serious killer survival threats as well as SAVE YOUR LIFE when you get in life or death situations. His trade secrets, Programs, and Videos are only offered to IRISAP subscribers-YOU!

- US Army Airborne School
- US Army Special Forces Qualification Course - SFQC (Green Beret)
- US Army Master Parachutist Wings
- Uruguayan Parachutist Wings
- British Parachutist Wings
- Kingdom of Jordan Parachutist Wings
- Expert Infantry Badge - EIB
- 82nd Airborne Division Recondo Course
- Adverse Weather Aerial Delivery System Tests - AWADS (01 of 386 volunteer paratroopers)
- US Army Special Forces Weapons Course (US & foreign pistols, submachineguns, assault rifles, rifles, machineguns, mortars, anti-tank weapons, anti-aircraft weapons,…)

- Weapons Armorer Course
- Indirect Fire Course (60mm, 81mm, & 4.2 inch *"four deuce"* mortars)
- Jumpmaster Course
- Basic French Language Course
- Combat Infantry Badge - CIB
- US Army Ranger Course
- Advanced Navigation Course
- Special Forces Sniper Course (02)
- Survival Evasion Resistance and Escape Instructor Course (SERE Level B)
- Wilderness Survival Instructor (College level - 03 years / 1991 - 1994)
- Rappell Master
- Fast Rope Master
- International Sniper Instructor
- International Close Quarter Battle (CQB) Instructor
- Participated In Multiple Combat Actions
- Special Forces Operations And Intelligence Course (O&I)
- Good Conduct Medal (06)
- Army Commendation Medal
- Army Achievement Medal (02)
- Meritorious Service Medal (02)
- Armed Forces Expeditionary Medal
- Letters Of Commendation (13)
- Letters Of Appreciation (08)
- Infantry Advanced NCO Course (11B)**
- Infantry Officer Basic Course **
- Military Intelligence Officer Basic Course **
- Held **SECRET** and **TOP SECRET Clearances** for 20+ years

** = These are military home study correspondence courses which took years to complete. This demonstrates Mr. Laydon's dedication to duty and desire to go beyond the training standards set by the US Army Special Forces. You won't find too many soldiers completing years of military home study courses on their own time off. This reflects the author's many superior Survival Products like this Survival Product.

Featured on FOX-2 (24 August 2000). Joseph now resides in Illinois. He offers products concerning Wilderness Survival, Health Survival, Crime Survival and Money Survival so to greatly enhance the lives of all IRISAP subscribers - YOU! Any questions, write to Joseph today.

Sincerely,
Joseph A. Laydon Jr. (IRISAP)
P.O. Box 48
Cutler, IL 62238-0048

You And Yours Have A Safe One
Anytime Anywhere,

Joseph A. Laydon Jr.

E-Mail: wwwsurvivalexpert@yahoo.com

E-Mail: josephlaydonjr@gmail.com

WEBSITES

- Main Website--------------------www.survivalexpert.com
- 45+ Survival Paperback Books-----www.survivalexpertbooks.com
- 45+ Survival Kindle E-Books------www.survivalexpertebooks.com
- Anytime Anywhere Survival--------www.anytimeanywheresurvival.com
- Weight-Loss---------------------www.loseitorelseweightloss.com
- True Scary Videos---------------www.patreon.com/truescaryvideos
- Exodus To Genesis (Fiction Book)-www.exodustogenesis.com
- **NEW** - 'Survival Expert Blog'--https://www.survivalexpertblog.com

Take Notes

Take Notes

Take Notes

Take Notes

Take Notes

Take Notes

More Super Healthy Survival Books Just For YOU!

Joseph A. Laydon Jr. (MSG Ret. Army) is the author and owner of Intensive Research Information Services And Products (IRISAP). Joseph has been writing *"self-reliance"* orientated data since 1991 and since July 2012 has been re-publishing his works via Kindle E-Books and CreateSpace Paperback Books. See *"About The Author."*

- **Kindle E-Books:**--------------------www.amazon.com (type title in Search Bar)

- **Paperback Books:**----------------- www.amazon.com (type title in Search Bar)

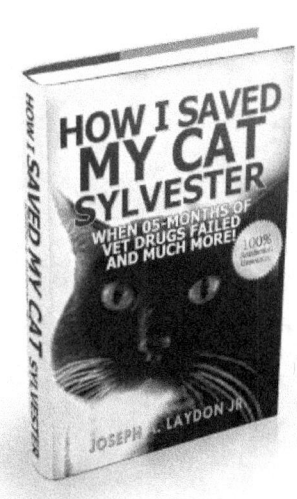 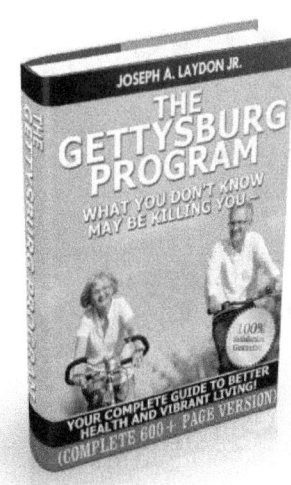

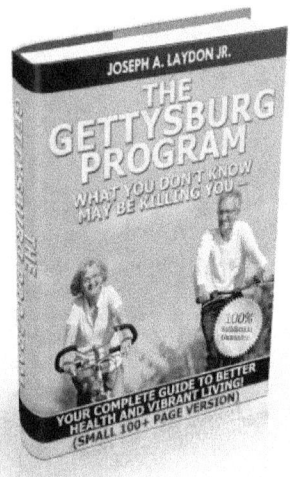

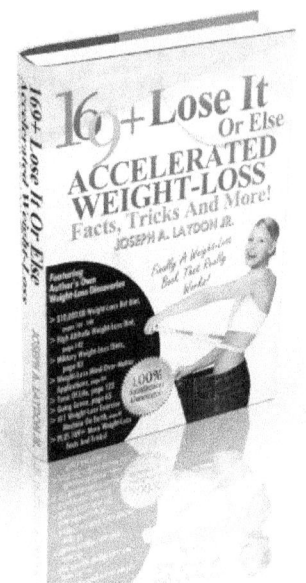

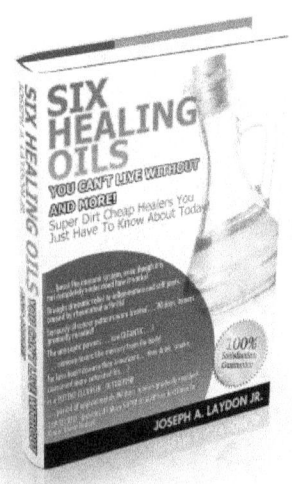

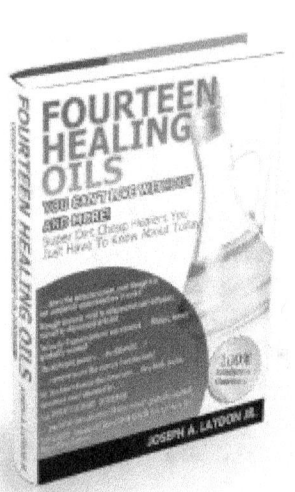

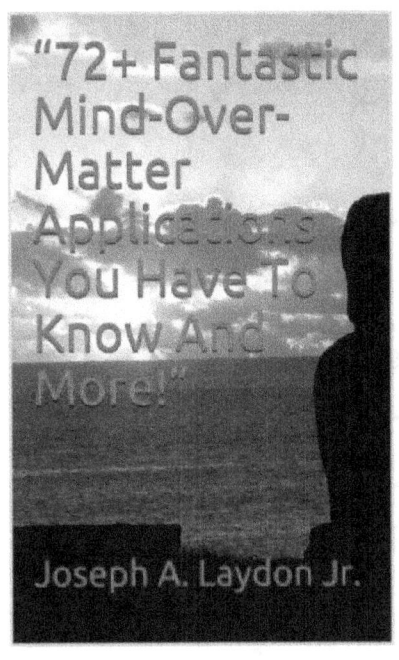

"72+ Fantastic Mind-Over-Matter Applications You Have To Know And More!"

Joseph A. Laydon Jr.

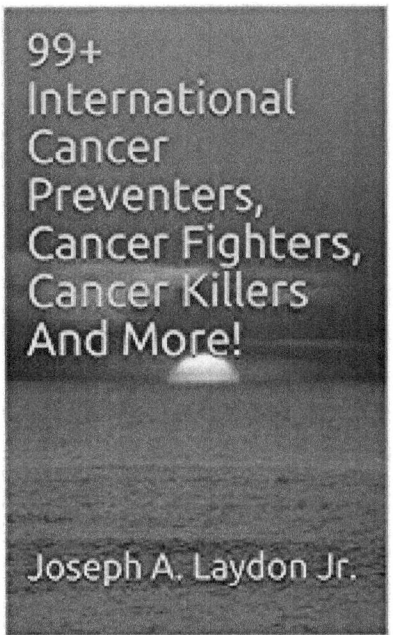

99+ International Cancer Preventers, Cancer Fighters, Cancer Killers And More!

Joseph A. Laydon Jr.

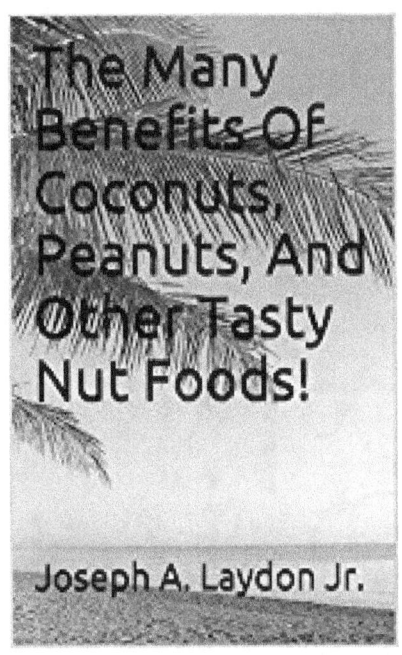

The Many Benefits Of Coconuts, Peanuts, And Other Tasty Nut Foods!

Joseph A. Laydon Jr.

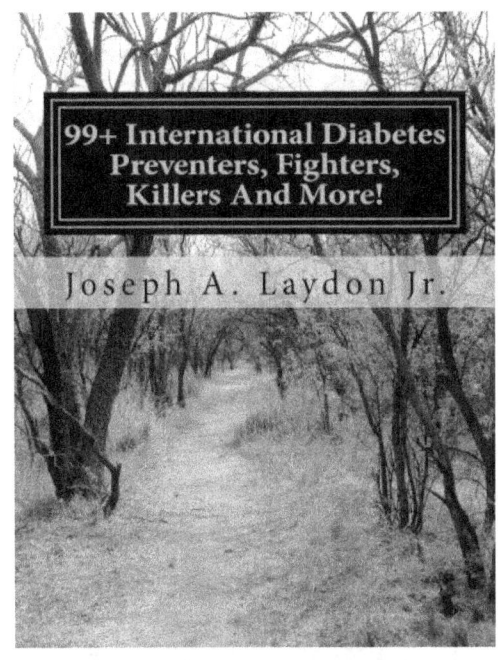

99+ International Diabetes Preventers, Fighters, Killers And More!

Joseph A. Laydon Jr.

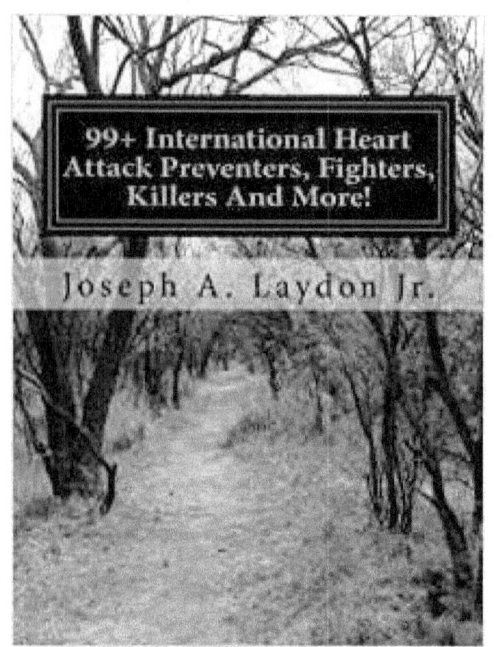

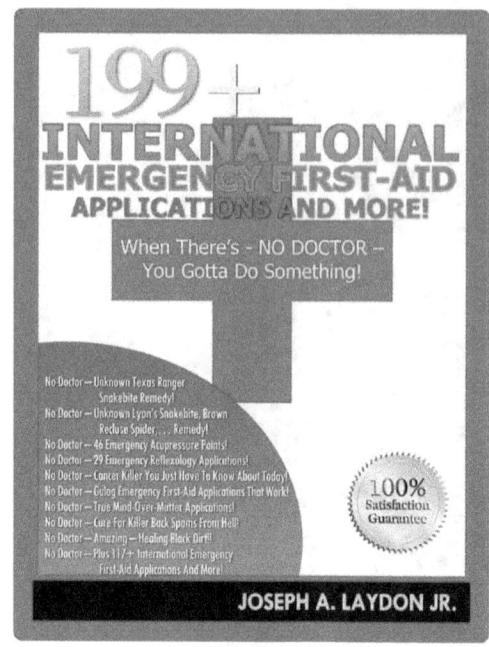

"Each Year 18,000 SAR Missions Are Looking For Lost People – 4,104 Are Found Too Late!"

LACK OF NAVIGATION has already killed multitudes of outdoor enthusiasts like:

- Bird Watchers
- Boaters
- Campers
- Fishermen
- Hikers
- Hunters
- Spelunkers
- Snowmobilers
- Treasure hunters

In the United States alone, **approximately 282 million people visit US National Parks** each year. There's an estimated 50,000 Search And Rescue (SAR) missions each year. And 18,000 of those SAR missions are looking for people who are lost in the wilderness!

And out of those 18,000 SAR missions looking for lost people in the wilderness, an estimated **4,104 are found too late** – they were killed by Mother Nature and all She possesses because of **LACK OF NAVIGATION!**

In the United States alone, there are **BILLIONS OF ACRES of wilderness land** (Federal, State and Private). I want you to get my *"Basic & Advanced Navigation Workbook And Videos!"* Home-Study Navigational Course below. If you don't, PLEASE learn how to navigate and carry & USE a map on all your outdoor adventures.

Basic & Advanced Navigation Workbook And Videos!

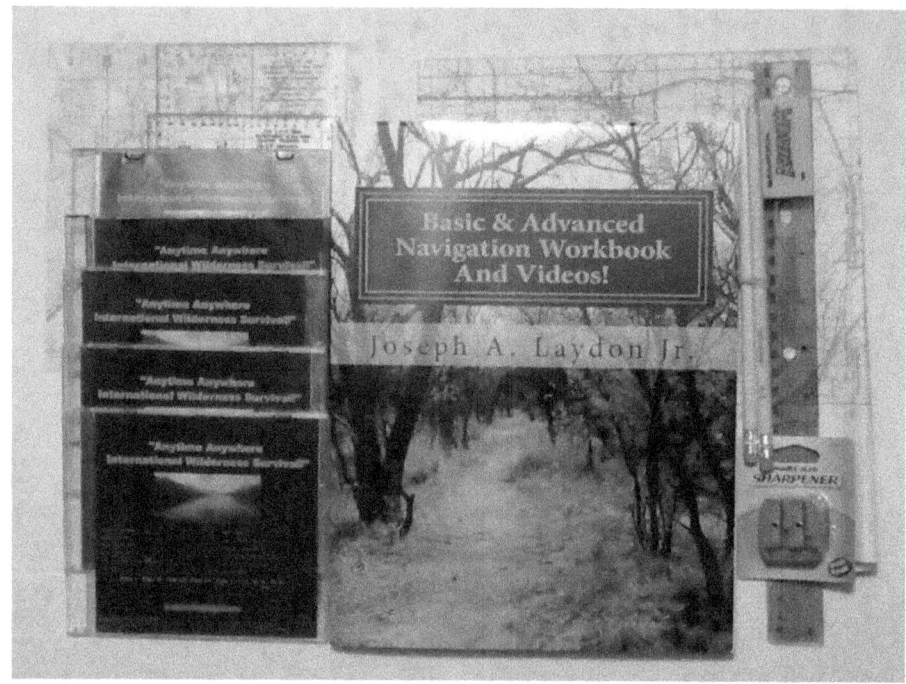

THANK YOU for getting this Survival Book. I appreciate your patronage. I thought you might be interested in this Survival Product. I'm not bragging – but it's a stone cold FACT! Here's one of the best navigation courses anywhere on Earth – *Basic & Advanced Navigation Workbook And Videos*. It's modeled after my 20-years in the US Army – namely the Special Forces (Green Berets).

Send Me Your Final Exam And I'll Send You A Set Of Long Range Walkie-Talkies!

If you venture outdoors (hunting, camping, hiking, fishing, rock-finding, rock climbing, Search And Rescue, military, law enforcement,…) **you absolutely have to know how to read a map and navigate cross country so you're in-control**. And even if you are lost, just by knowing how to read a map, you can '*find yourself*' instead of becoming completely lost leading to another '*dead statistic.*'

In this navigation course, I'll start you at the very basics in map reading. Do this: take your index finger and draw a circle in the air in front of you. Go ahead and draw a circle. Good. That circle you just drew represents a hill top. A hill top on any map anywhere on the Earth.

That's how I start teaching you how to read maps. We start at the very basics. Then we   s l o w l y   progress into the military grid system. You ever see those maps with bunches of squares all over the map – that's the military grid system. We'll start out at the baby level and work up reading 04-digit grid coordinates, 06-digit grid coordinates and then 08-digit grid coordinates. I give you spot quizzes here and throughout the entire Workbook. And all the answers are already in the book so you can check your work.

After you do all the military grid system problems, then we'll transition into GEO Coordinates. GEO Coordinates means Geographical Coordinates of Latitude, Longitude – Degrees, Minutes, and Seconds. You'll be able to plot and find GEO Coordinates anywhere on Earth. You'll be one of the few people on Earth that can read and plot military grid coordinates and GEO Coordinates.

And here's the reason you're going to be one of the best navigators on Earth. The Workbook and the 06+ hours of Videos are synced together. As you go through page by page in the workbook, you'll see everything in the videos. To make sure you understand everything, I give you spot quizzes after each seqment, each section. And all the answers are in the Workbook so you can check your work. If you have any concerns, just review the videos.

And I provide you with everything you need to do all the navigational problems (see list below).

- **Basic Map Reading DVD Video:** Basic Map Reading DVD Video (02:03:19). View this video and do some of the navigational problems before you start the main course. This DVD Video comes with a color map.

- **Field-Expedient Direction DVD Video:** Field-Expedient Direction DVD Video (02:02:45)

  View this video a couple times before you start the main course. You'll learn alternative ways to find direction anywhere on Earth when you have no compass or you're verifying your compass heading).

Basic & Advanced Navigation Workbook And Videos!

- **Basic and Advanced Navigation Workbook:** Basic and Advanced Navigation Workbook clocks-in at 300-pages with a word count of 41,152. This Workbook has hundreds of time hacks throughout the book that are synced to all the DVD Videos. It has explanations and sketches and 440 practice navigational problems and all the answers are in the Workbook so you can check your own answers.

- **Basic and Advanced Navigation Workbook DVD Videos:** You get multiple DVD Videos (06:30:00) that are synched to the Navigation Workbook. Basic and Advanced Navigation And all these

- **02 Full Large Tenino Maps Sheets:** You'll get 02 full large Tenino Map Sheets. Use the 1st map for all your work. Use the 1st map for all the Spot Quizzes and Practice Final Exam. Use the 2nd map for the Final Exam. Send it in to me with your answers and scratch paper so I can see you did all your work and I'll send you a set of long-range Walkie-Talkies (keep reading).

- **02 Military Protractors:** You'll get 02 military protractors (01 back-up protractor). The military protractor is used to plot grid azimuths on your maps and to plot 06-digit & 08-digit Grid Coordinates. Don't worry, I'll explain everything in the DVD videos.

- **02 Pencils, Pencil Sharpener & Gum Erasers:** I told you I'll send you everything for the *Basic & Advanced Navigation Workbook And Videos*. You'll have 02 pencils, a pencil sharpener for drawing thin lines, and 02 gum erasers in case you make some mistakes.

- **02 Rulers:** The transparent 12-inch ruler (01 back-up ruler) is used to draw your grid azimuth lines across your maps and it's also used to plot your GEO Coordinates of Latitude and Longitude - Degrees, Minutes, and Seconds on the Tenino Maps or any other map. I'll explain everything in the DVD videos.

- **Basic And Advanced Navigation Practice Final Exam:** You're almost done. You've done plenty of navigational problems, now you're ready for the Practice Final Exam. Included in the Navigation Workbook is a Practice Final Exam. And guess what? All the answers are in the Workbook so you can check your own work! Once you pass the Practice Final Exam, you're 110% ready for the Final Exam.

- **Basic And Advanced Navigation Final Exam:** BIG CONGRATS!!! You made it this far. You already passed your Practice Final Exam, now you're ready for the Final Exam. Hey, take a day or two off and recharge your batteries. Odds are 110% that when you pass the Practice Final Exam, **you will pass** the Final Exam. And to MOTIVATE you to take the Final Exam and pass it, I'll send you a set of long-range Walkie-Talkies with back-up batteries - FREE!

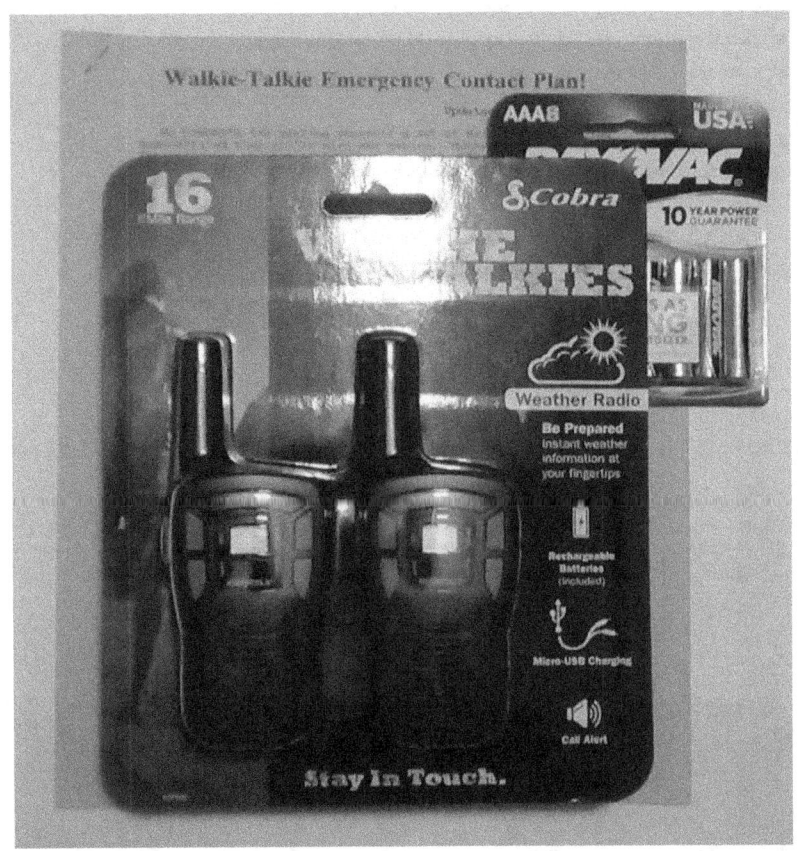

Pass the *Basic And Advanced Navigation Final Exam* and I'll send you:
- A set of Long Range Walkie-Talkies
- Walkie-Talkie Emergency Contact Plan
- Back-Up Batteries

The reason I want to send you a set of Walkie-Talkies is because when you're venturing outdoors (NEVER go alone), **communications** will PREVENT outdoor tragedies and REMEDY outdoor tragedies. On the next page is your Order Form to get the *Basic & Advanced Navigation Workbook And Videos*.

"Basic & Advanced Navigation Workbook And Videos!" Order Form Certificate

EASY INSTRUCTIONS: Read and CUT-OUT this entire Order Form Certificate. It authorizes you to get your own *"Basic & Advanced Navigation Workbook And Videos!"* CUT-OUT and Fill-in this Order Form Certificate. Return to IRISAP today. You'll get:

- **Basic Map Reading DVD Video** (02:03:19)
- **Field-Expedient Direction DVD Video** (02:02:45)
- **Basic and Advanced Navigation Workbook** (300-pages)
- **Basic and Advanced Navigation Workbook DVD Videos** (06:30:00)
- **02 Full Large Tenino Maps Sheets**
- **02 Military Protractors**
- **02 Pencils, Pencil Sharpener & 02 Gum Erasers**
- **02 Rulers**
- **Basic And Advanced Navigation Practice Final Exam**
- **Basic And Advanced Navigation Final Exam**

YES, get your own *"Basic & Advanced Navigation Workbook And Videos!"* I confidently give you a 01-Year Money-Back Guarantee and a After 01-Year DOUBLE Money-Back Guarantee! I KNOW you'll say: *"BEST investment I ever made!"* REMEMBER, You Get My Personal NO RISK UNCONDITIONAL *"01-Year Money-Back Guarantee and NO RISK UNCONDITIONAL After 01-Year DOUBLE Money-Back Guarantee!"*

"Basic & Advanced Navigation Workbook And Videos!"

OK, YES OF COURSE - Joseph, I'll fill-in the data below. I have a UNCONDITIONAL NO RISK 01-Year Money Back Guarantee & A UNCONDITIONAL After 01-Year DOUBLE Money-Back Guarantee! Joseph, I don't want to get lost and be another DEAD STATISTIC - so here's my order and payment of $389.97 plus $19.00 for postage & handling - total **$408.97**:

Name:_____
        Sign full name I'm OVER 21 YEARS OF AGE (17+ years waived to active duty military)

_____$408.97 full payment (**Money Orders** get Priority Processing)
Foreign Orders MUST ADD $39.00 for Priority Mail Postage (total $447.97).

Full Name:_____
      (Last)   (First)   (MI)   (Jr. Sn. I, II, III)

Address:_____

City:_____ State:_____ Zip:_____

Country:_____

Phone Number:_____
      (Area Code)   (I'll only call if there is a delay with your order)

SEND ORDER FORM and PAYMENT TO:
Joseph A. Laydon Jr. (IRISAP - NAV 1)
P.O. Box 48
Cutler, IL 62238-0048
United States of America
E-Mail: wwwsurvivalexpert@yahoo.com